DEVELOPING A WORLD CLASS
CLINICAL TRIAL SITE

DEVELOPING A WORLD CLASS
CLINICAL TRIAL SITE

A STEP BY STEP GUIDE TO BE A
SUCCESSFUL CLINICAL TRIAL SITE

Dr. P.K. Julka

CR Books

First Published in India by
CR Books Pvt. Ltd.
503, Block-C, NDM-2, Netaji Subhash Place, Pitampura, Delhi-110034 (India)
Tel: 011-45121445 Fax: 011-45121435
E-mail: info@crbooks.in, info@crbooks.us
Web: www.crbooks.net

First Edition: August 2011
Second Edition: June 2014

The author and publisher have made a conscientious effort to ensure that the
information contained in this book is accurate and in accordance with the
accepted standards at the time of publication. However, in this
rapidly changing world guidelines and practices are subject
to change without prior notification, therefore readers are
advised to confirm these as and when needed.

Typeset in Calibri by
nadeem.anees@gmail.com

ISBN 81-922277-3-3

Contents

Appendices

Preface

Internationally, India became a member of World Trade Organization (WTO) in 1995 and agreed to adhere to the product patent regime from year 2005 onwards. As a result, global pharmaceutical industry has the rights to patent product as well as processes throughout the world, including India. As a signatory of WTO Agreements, India is being looked upon as a favorable destination for conducting global clinical trials.

Data suggests a 50-60% cost saving by conducting clinical trials in India compared to the same clinical trials being conducted in the U.S. or Western Europe. This is evident by a steadily increasing number of global clinical trials in India over past few years. It is estimated that more than 4500 clinical trials are being conducted in India across 5000+ investigator sites and there is a growing need of newer investigator sites.

This book is intended to provide an insight on becoming a successful clinical trial investigator. While navigating through the book, a reader would be able to develop a clear understanding on the steps involved in developing a good clinical trial site.

The first edition of this book was very well appreciated by various clinical trial stakeholders. An updated information in certain sections have been incorporated in the current edition. I hope this edition will leave the desired impression and readers would be able to incorporate the learnings in to the practice.

Dr. P. K. Julka

1

Introduction to Clinical Research

Clinical research refers to a systematic investigation in human subjects for evaluating the safety and efficacy of any new drug. In today's scientific era research is taking a major stride in all streams and newer and better drugs are being introduced to cure ailments, which are difficult to treat. Clinical trials are the mainstay for bringing out new drugs to the market and constitute approximately 70% of the total time and money spent in drug discovery process. Typically it takes approximately 12 years and US$ 1 billion to bring one new drug from conception to market out of which 6-7 years are spent in various phases of clinical trials. Before studying clinical research, it is important to understand the overall drug discovery process.

1.1 Drug Discovery Process

The drug discovery process begins with the generation of a new idea that is targeted towards chemically modifying a disease process via a drug. The idea is usually generated from a comprehensive understanding of a disease process and a continuing involvement with research in specific therapeutic area of interest. The first step is selection and validation of a 'Target' which is followed by selection of 'Drug' that has the ability to interact with the Target.

> ➤ Target selection involves choosing a disease to treat and then developing a model for that disease. Thus researcher first select or discover a biological target such as a particular enzyme, receptor or ion channel that the scientific team believes may be linked to a pathological process. It is estimated that up to 10 genes

contribute to multi-factorial diseases[1]. These disease genes are further linked to another 5 to 10 gene product in physiological and pathophysiological pathways leading to an availability of approximately 10,000 potential drug targets.

➢ Target validation involves demonstration of relevance of the target protein in a disease process.

➢ Drug selection or Lead selection is a process that involves finding a drug or group of drugs which has the ability to interact with target protein and modulate its activity. Tens of thousands of potential drug substances (obtained from massive compound libraries) are tested against the target proteins in a robotic process called High Throughput Screening (HTS).

➢ HTS yields Hit compounds that are further studied in detail for their physical, chemical and biological properties. Hit compounds with suitable physical, chemical and biological properties are called Lead candidates.

➢ Lead Candidates are then chemically modified and pharmacologically characterized to obtain compounds with suitable pharmacodynamic and pharmacokinetic properties to become a drug in a process called Lead optimization.

The compound with best profile is then chosen for further investigation in the form of preclinical and clinical testing.

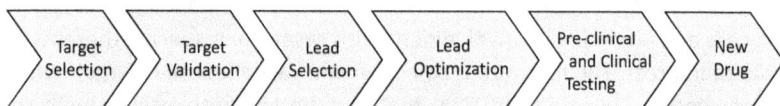

Target Selection > Target Validation > Lead Selection > Lead Optimization > Pre-clinical and Clinical Testing > New Drug

Figure 1. Drug Discovery Process

1.2 Preclinical Testing

Preclinical tests are performed in the laboratory, using a wide array of chemical and biochemical assays, cell-culture models and animal models. The pharmacological activity of every new compound is carefully analyzed.

As the experience with the compound increases, experimental steps and methods can be modified. Preclinical testing involves:

➤ Pharmacological testing

➤ Toxicology testing (acute, sub-acute, chronic, reproductive and mutagenic)

➤ Animal pharmacokinetic testing

1.3 Clinical Testing

Clinical testing of a drug is done in four phases (I, II, III and IV) of clinical trials. The knowledge gained from one phase is assessed before progressing to the next phase. However, research in a particular phase may continue after the drug has progressed to further stages of development.

Phase-I clinical trials are conducted to establish initial safety, maximum tolerance and pharmacokinetics of a new drug in 20-80 healthy human volunteers (with the exception of cancer drugs where Phase-I trials are done on cancer patients). These are also called as 'First in Man' and acts as a basis of validating the findings from pre-clinical testing in to human beings. Usually Phase-I trials are initiated with a very low dose (1/10th of the optimal animal dose) which is gradually increased to determine the maximum tolerated dose. During Phase-I trials, sufficient information about the drug's pharmacokinetics and pharmacological effects is obtained to plan a well-controlled, Phase-II trial.

An Investigational New Drug (IND) Application is filed to regulatory authorities for seeking the permission to initiate Phase-I clinical trials.

Phase-II clinical trials are universally accepted as a standard requirement for the evaluation of efficacy and safety of a new drug. Careful observations are made to determine the dose and adverse reactions in 100-200 patients with the relevant indication. If a new drug is found to be effective and safe in Phase-II trials, it is moved to next phase of development. In case of lack of efficacy the development of drug is stopped at this phase itself.

Phase-III clinical trials are the final pre-marketing phase of clinical trials.

These are large, multi-centric trials to establish the safety and efficacy of a new drug *vis-à-vis* existing standard of care/placebo that forms the basis for regulatory submission. If a new drug is found to be safe and effective in Phase-III trials, a New Drug Application (NDA) is filed to regulatory authorities for seeking marketing permission.

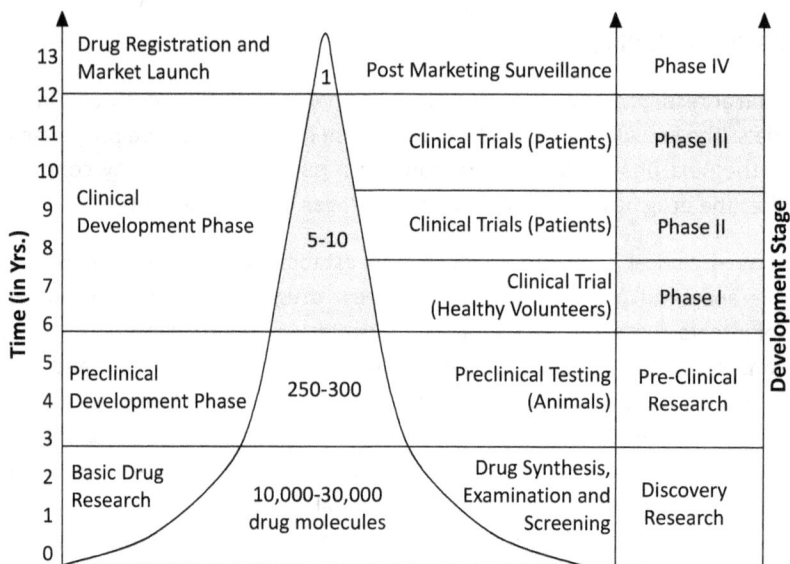

Time (in Yrs.)			Development Stage	
13	Drug Registration and Market Launch	1	Post Marketing Surveillance	Phase IV
12				
11			Clinical Trials (Patients)	Phase III
10				
9	Clinical Development Phase	5-10	Clinical Trials (Patients)	Phase II
8				
7			Clinical Trial (Healthy Volunteers)	Phase I
6				
5	Preclinical Development Phase	250-300	Preclinical Testing (Animals)	Pre-Clinical Research
4				
3				
2	Basic Drug Research	10,000-30,000 drug molecules	Drug Synthesis, Examination and Screening	Discovery Research
1				
0				

Figure 2. Drug Development Process

Phase-IV clinical trials are post marketing studies that are conducted for generating additional safety data on a drug once it is marketed. Regulatory authorities can withdraw the marketing authorization of a drug anytime if there are safety concerns on its usage.

It is estimated that for every 10,000-30,000 drug molecules screened; only 250-300 enters the pre-clinical testing, 5 enters the clinical testing and 1 reaches to the market.

4

```
        ┌─────────┐
        │   IND   │
        └─────────┘
             ↓
         Phase-I
         Phase-II
         Phase-III
             ↓
        ┌─────────┐
        │   NDA   │
        └─────────┘
             ↓
 ┌──────────────────────────┐
 │  Marketing Authorization │
 └──────────────────────────┘
```

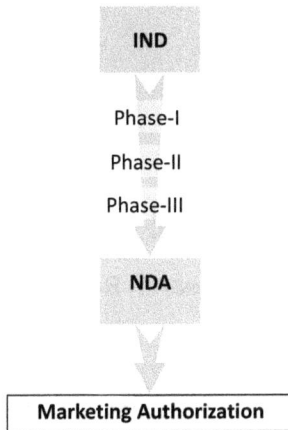

Figure 3. Drug Approval Process

Summary Points

☑ Drug Discovery and Development Process involves target selection, target validation, drug/lead selection, lead optimization, pre-clinical and clinical testing.

☑ Clinical trials refer to a systematic investigation in human subjects for evaluating the safety and efficacy of any new drug.

☑ Clinical trials are the mainstay for bringing out new drugs to the market.

☑ Clinical trials are done in four phases (phase I, II, III and IV).

☑ It is estimated that for every 10,000-30,000 drug molecules screened only 1 reaches to the market.

☑ It takes approximately 12 years and US$ 1 billion to bring one new drug to the market.

References:

1. Drews J. Drug Discovery: a historical perspective. Science 2000; 287: 1960-64.

2

Clinical Research Regulations

The present day ethical research principles, regulations and guidelines have evolved over a period of time after a series of scientific misconduct/fraud. Prior to World War II there was very little concern for the participation of human subjects in medical research and therefore there was no formal protection. It started with Nuremberg Code in 1947, the same year when the World Medical Association (WMA) was established.

2.1 Nuremberg Code[1]

In 1947 the Nuremberg Code laid down 10 principles to guide physician investigators for experiments involving human subjects. The need to define the basic principles for the conduct of human research was focused towards patient protection and made no distinctions between research with patient-subjects and healthy persons, be they prisoners or volunteers. The Nuremberg Code was the result of judgment by an American military war crimes tribunal conducting proceedings against 23 Nazi physicians and administrators for their wilful participation in war crimes and crimes against humanity. The doctors had conducted medical experiments on concentration camp prisoners who died or were permanently affected as a result. The Nuremberg Code was developed in response to the judicial condemnation of the acts of Nazi physicians, and did not specifically address human subject research in the context of the patient-physician relationship.

The 10 principles of the Nuremberg Code are as follows:

1.   The voluntary free consent to participate;

2. The experiment to yield fruitful results for the good of society, unprocurable by other methods or means of study;

3. The experiment should be designed based on the results of animal experimentation or other previous work;

4. The experiment should avoid all unnecessary physical and mental suffering and injury;

5. No experiment should be conducted where there is an a priori reason to believe that death or disabling injury will occur;

6. The degree of risk to be taken should never exceed that determined by experiment;

7. Proper preparations should be made to protect the experimental subject against even remote possibilities of injury, disability, or death;

8. The research study should be conducted only by scientifically qualified persons;

9. Participants can withdraw from the study at any time;

10. Cessation of study if adverse effects emerges

2.2 Declaration of Helsinki[2]

The World Medial Association (WMA) has developed the Declaration of Helsinki as a statement of ethical principles to provide guidance to physicians and other participants in medical research involving human subjects.

Declaration of Helsinki was adopted by the 18th WMA General Assembly, Helsinki, Finland, June 1964 and amended by the 29th WMA General Assembly, Tokyo, Japan, October 1975; 35th WMA General Assembly, Venice, Italy, October 1983; 41st WMA General Assembly, Hong Kong, September 1989; 48th WMA General Assembly, Somerset West, Republic of South Africa, October 1996; 52nd WMA General Assembly, Edinburgh, Scotland, October 2000, 59th WMA General Assembly, Seoul, October 2008 and 64th WMA General Assembly, Fortaleza, Brazil, October 2013.

The Declaration of Geneva of the WMA binds the physician with the words, "The health of my patient will be my first consideration", and the

International Code of Medical Ethics declares that, "A physician shall act only in the patient's interest when providing medical care which might have the effect of weakening the physical and mental condition of the patient". Declaration of Helsinki laid down the Ethical Principles for Medical Research Involving Human Subject and is a major landmark in the evolution of Good Clinical Practices (GCPs).

The basic principles of the Declaration of Helsinki include the following:

- Physician's duty in research is to protect the life, health, privacy, and dignity of the human participant
- Research involving humans must conform to generally accepted scientific principles and thorough knowledge of scientific literature and methods
- Research protocols should be reviewed by an independent committee
- Research protocols should be conducted by medically/scientifically qualified individuals
- Risks and burden to the participant should not outweigh benefits
- Researcher should stop study if risks are found to outweigh potential benefits
- Research is justified only if there is a reasonable likelihood that the population under study will benefit from the results
- Participation must be voluntary and through a written consent
- Every precaution must be taken to respect privacy, confidentiality, and participant's physical and mental integrity
- Assent must be obtained from minors
- Investigators are obliged to preserve the accuracy of results; negative and positive results should be publicly available

2.3 The Belmont Report, 1979[3]

The Belmont Report, created by the former United States Department of Health, Education and Welfare is an important historical document in the field of medical ethics. The report was created on April 18, 1979 and gets its name from the Belmont Conference Center where the document was drafted.

The Belmont Report explains the unifying ethical principles that form the basis for the National Commission's topic-specific reports and the regulations that incorporate its recommendations. The three fundamental ethical principles for using any human subject for research are:

1. Respect for Persons: protecting the autonomy of all people and treating them with courtesy and respect and allowing for informed consent,

2. Beneficence: maximizing benefits for the research project while minimizing risks to the research subjects,

3. Justice: ensuring reasonable, non-exploitative and well considered procedures are administered fairly (the fair distribution of costs and benefits to potential research participants).

The applications of 1, 2, and 3, respectively, are informed consent, assessment of risks and benefits, and selection of subjects.

2.4 ICH - Good Clinical Practice (GCP) of 1997[4]

The Food and Drug Administration (FDA) has published guidelines entitled "Good Clinical Practice: Consolidated Guideline". The guideline was prepared under the auspices of the International Conference on Harmonization of Technical Requirements for Registration of Pharmaceuticals for Human Use (ICH). The guideline is intended to define "Good Clinical Practice" and to provide a unified ethical and scientific quality standard for designing, conducting, recording and reporting trials that involve the participation of human subjects. Compliance with this standard provides public assurance that the rights, safety and well being of trial subjects are protected, consistent with the principles that have their origin in the Declaration of Helsinki, and that the clinical trial data are credible.

The objective of the ICH-GCP Guidelines is to provide a unified standard for the European Union (EU), Japan and the United States to facilitate the mutual acceptance of clinical data by the regulatory authorities in these jurisdictions. The guideline was developed with consideration of the current good clinical practices of the European Union, Japan, and the United States, as well as those of Australia, Canada, the Nordic countries and the World Health Organization (WHO). These guidelines are required to be followed while generating clinical trial data that is intended to be submitted to regulatory authorities. The principles established in this guideline may also be applied to other clinical investigations that may have an impact on the safety and well-being of human subjects.

The Principles of GCP

1. Clinical trials should be conducted in accordance with the ethical principles that have their origin in the Declaration of Helsinki, and that are consistent with GCP and the applicable regulatory requirement(s).

2. Before a trial is initiated, foreseeable risks and inconveniencies should be weighed against the anticipated benefit for the individual trial subject and society. A trial should be initiated and continued only if the anticipated benefits justify the risks.

3. The rights, safety, and well being of the trial subjects are the most important considerations and should prevail over interests of science and society.

4. The available non-clinical and clinical information on an investigational product should be adequate to support the proposed clinical trial.

5. Clinical trials should be scientifically sound, and described in a clear, detailed protocol.

6. A trial should be conducted in compliance with the protocol that has received prior institutional review board (IRB)/independent ethics committee (IEC) approval/favourable opinion.

7. The medical care given to, and medical decisions made on behalf of, subjects should always be the responsibility of a qualified physician or, when appropriate, of a qualified dentist.

8. Each individual involved in conducting a trial should be qualified by education, training, and experience to perform his or her respective task(s).

9. Freely given informed consent should be obtained from every subject prior to clinical trial participation.

10. All clinical trial information should be recorded, handled, and stored in a way that allows its accurate reporting, interpretation, and verification.

11. The confidentiality of records that could identify subjects should be protected, respecting the privacy and confidentiality rules in accordance with the applicable regulatory requirement(s).

12. Investigational products should be manufactured, handled, and stored in accordance with applicable good manufacturing practice (GMP). They should be used in accordance with the approved protocol.

13. System with procedures that assure the quality of every aspect of the trials should be implemented.

2.5 Ethical Guidelines for Biomedical Research on Human Subjects, 2006 (ICMR Code)[5]

Indian Council of Medical Research, New Delhi has issued the statement of Ethical Guidelines for Biomedical Research on Human Subjects also known ICMR Code, in the year 2000. Revised guidelines were released in the year 2006. These guidelines include statement of general and specific principles on research using human subjects in biomedical research. The statement of general principles include following principles:

➤ Principles of essentiality

➤ Principles of voluntariness, informed consent and community agreement

➤ Principles of non-exploitation

➤ Principles of privacy and confidentiality

➤ Principles of precaution and risk minimization

➤ Principles of professional competence

➤ Principles of accountability and transparency

- Principles of the maximization of the public interest and of distributive justice
- Principles of institutional arrangements
- Principles of public domain
- Principles of totality of responsibilities
- Principles of compliance

The statement of specific principles includes guidelines for clinical evaluation of drugs, vaccines, devices, diagnostics and herbal remedies etc.

2.6 Good Clinical Practices, 2001 (Indian GCP)[6]

These guidelines for clinical trials on pharmaceutical products in India have been evolved with consideration of WHO, ICH, USFDA and European GCP guidelines as well as the Ethical Guidelines for Biomedical Research on Human Subjects issued by the Indian Council of Medical Research (ICMR).

The Drug Technical Advisory Board (DTAB), the highest technical body under Drugs and Cosmetic Act, has endorsed adoption of these GCP guidelines for streamlining the clinical studies in India. These guidelines should be followed for carrying out all biomedical research in India at all stages of drug development, whether prior or subsequent to product registration in India.

2.7 Schedule-Y[7]

Schedule-Y of Drugs and Cosmetics Act 1940 detail the requirements and guidelines for permission to import and/or manufacture of new drugs for sale or to undertake clinical trials.

In India, a two tier regulatory approval process is followed:

1. Trial approval at individual site level by the respective ethics committee
2. Trial approval at country level by office of DCGI

Ethics committee approval from at least one site is generally required in order to apply for regulatory approval.

```
┌─────────────────────────────┐
│       Trial Proposal        │
└─────────────────────────────┘
              ↓
┌─────────────────────────────────────────┐
│  Ethics Approval at Individual Site Level │
└─────────────────────────────────────────┘
              ↓
┌─────────────────────────────────────────────┐
│       DCGI Approval at Country Level          │
│  (Trial Permission, import/export licenses)   │
└─────────────────────────────────────────────┘
              ↓
         Trial Initiation
```

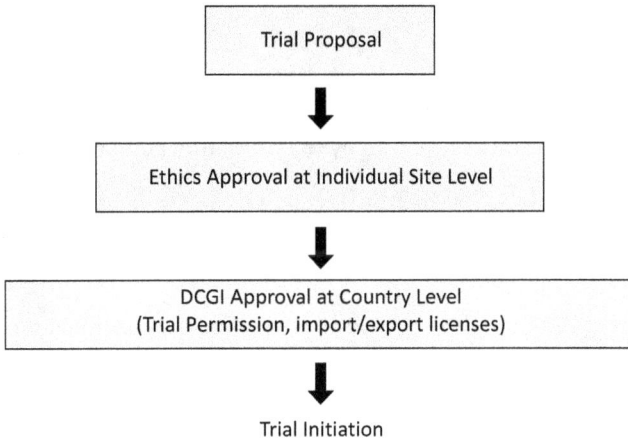

Figure 4. Regulatory Approval Process

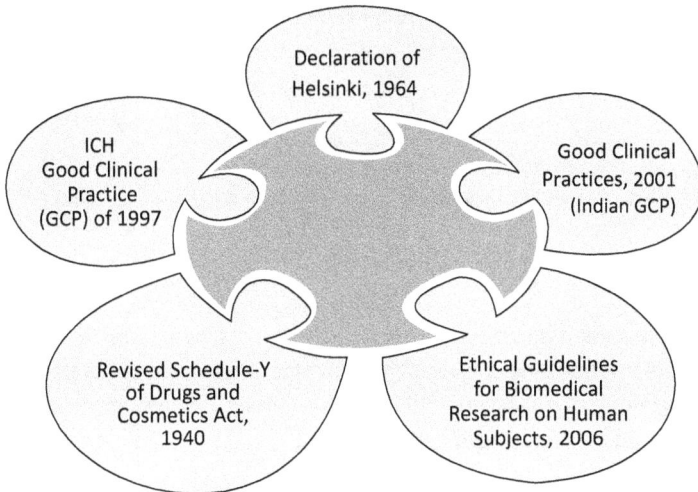

Declaration of Helsinki, 1964

ICH Good Clinical Practice (GCP) of 1997

Good Clinical Practices, 2001 (Indian GCP)

Revised Schedule-Y of Drugs and Cosmetics Act, 1940

Ethical Guidelines for Biomedical Research on Human Subjects, 2006

Figure 5. Clinical Research Regulations for the Conduct of Global Clinical Trials in India

Summary Points

☑ ICH-GCP Guidelines provide a unified standard for the European Union (EU), Japan and the United States to facilitate the mutual acceptance of clinical data by the regulatory authorities in these jurisdictions.

☑ ICMR Code includes statement of general and specific principles on research using human subjects in biomedical research.

☑ Indian GCP Guidelines have been evolved with consideration of WHO, ICH, USFDA and European GCP guidelines as well as ICMR Code.

☑ Schedule-Y of Drugs and Cosmetics Act 1940 detail the requirement and guidelines on clinical trials for import and manufacture of a new drug in India.

☑ The office of Drug Controller General of India (DCGI) under CDSCO has the prime responsibility for regulating Clinical trials in India.

References:

1. Trials of War Criminals before the Nuremberg Military Tribunals under Control Council Law No. 10, Vol. 2, pp. 181-182. Washington, D.C.: U.S. Government Printing Office, 1949.

2. World Medical Association Declaration of Helsinki, Ethical Principles for Medical Research Involving Human Subjects, Adopted by the 18th WMA General Assembly Helsinki, Finland, June 1964 and its subsequent amendments. Available from: http://www.wma.net/e/policy/b3.htm

3. Belmont Report (1979). Available from: http://www.hhs.gov/ohrp/humansubjects/guidance/belmont.html

4. http://www.ich.org [homepage on the Internet]: E6 (R1): Switzerland: Good Clinical Practice: Consolidated Guidelines. Available from: http://www.ich.org/LOB/media/MEDIA482.pdf

5. Ethical Guidelines for Biomedical Research on Human Subjects, Indian Council of Medical Research, 2006.

6.   Good Clinical Practices For Clinical Research In India. Available from: http://www.cdsco.nic.in/html/GCP1.html

7. Schedule-Y (Amended Version 2005). Available from: http://www.cdsco.nic.in/html/GCP1.html

3

Clinical Trial Stakeholders

Clinical Research is a team effort and requires involvement of various stakeholders to achieve the planned endpoint. Each stakeholder has a defined role and success can not be accomplished without involving individual stakeholder.

The various stakeholders include:

➢ Sponsor/ Contract Research Organization (CRO)

➢ Investigator

➢ Ethics Committee (EC)

➢ Regulatory Authority (*e.g.* FDA in US, DCGI in India *etc.*)

➢ Patients/Study Subjects

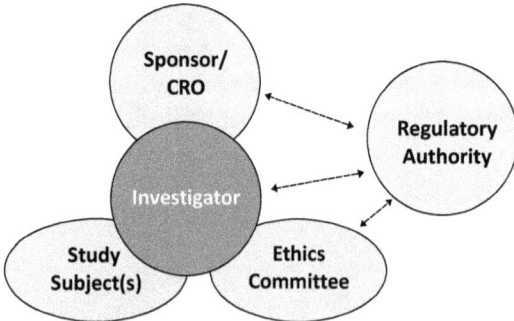

Figure 6. Clinical Trial Stakeholders

3.1 Sponsor/CRO

Sponsor refers to an individual, company, institution, or organization which takes responsibility for the initiation, management, and/or financing of a clinical trial.

Contract Research Organization (CRO) refers to a person or an organization (commercial, academic, or other) contracted by the sponsor to perform one or more of a sponsor's trial-related duties and functions.

The chief responsibilities of Sponsor/CRO are:

➢ Trial planning, development of essential trial documents and allocation of resources

➢ Logistics planning and appointment of central lab, CRO and other vendors

➢ Manufacturing and accountability of investigational product

➢ Investigator's selection and site set-up

➢ Regulatory submission and obtaining trial approval, import/export licenses

➢ Conducting investigator's training meeting

➢ Clinical trial monitoring

➢ Data management

➢ Pharmacovigilance

➢ Ensuring compliance with protocol, GCP and applicable regulatory guidelines

➢ Clinical trial auditing/quality assurance

➢ Preparation of clinical study report

➢ Trial closure

➢ Publication of trial results

➢ Obtaining marketing approval

3.2 Investigator

Investigator refers to a person who is responsible for the conduct of a clinical trial at a site.

The chief responsibilities of a clinical trial investigator are:

- ➤ Site organization and constitution of study team
- ➤ Delegation of responsibilities at site
- ➤ Submission of trial document to ethics committee and obtaining approval
- ➤ Trial initiation at site
- ➤ Administration of informed consent to study subjects
- ➤ Medical care of study subjects
- ➤ Source data documentation
- ➤ Medical record maintenance
- ➤ Drug dispensing and accountability
- ➤ Ensuring compliance with protocol, GCP and applicable regulatory guidelines
- ➤ Management of adverse events
- ➤ Reporting of serious adverse events to sponsor and ethics committee
- ➤ Communication with ethics committee and sponsor/CRO
- ➤ Site closure

3.3 Ethics Committee

Ethics committee refers to an independent body, constituted of medical professionals and non-medical members, whose responsibility is to ensure the protection of the rights, safety and well being of human subjects involved in a clinical trial and to provide public assurance of that protection by among other things, reviewing and approving/providing favorable opinion on, the trial protocol, the suitability of the investigator(s), facilities, and the methods and material to be used in obtaining and documenting informed consent of the trial subjects. Ethics committee is also called as Institutional Review Board (IRB), Institutional Ethics Committee (IEC) and Ethics Review Board (ERB).

The chief responsibilities of Ethics Committee are:

- ➤ Constitution and organization of ethics committee
- ➤ Review and approval of trial documents
- ➤ Meeting 'quorum' requirements
- ➤ Maintaining minutes of ethics meetings
- ➤ Review of protocol violations, adverse events/serious adverse events and periodic reports
- ➤ Ensuring compliance with GCP and applicable regulatory guidelines

3.4 Regulatory Authority

Regulatory authority refers to the drug control authorities or Food and Drug Administrations that have the authority to regulate.

The chief responsibilities of Regulatory Authority are:

- ➤ Laying down the rules and regulations
- ➤ Review of trial documents and granting trial permission/approval
- ➤ Review of protocol violations, adverse events/serious adverse events and periodic reports
- ➤ Termination/suspension of trial (if deemed appropriate)
- ➤ Inspection (Sponsor, CRO, Investigator, IRB/EC/IEC *etc.*)

3.5 Study Subject

Study subject refers to an individual who participates in a clinical trial.

The chief responsibilities of Study subject are:

- ➢ Voluntary consent for participation in a clinical trial
- ➢ Compliance with protocol schedule of events

Summary Points

- ☑ Stakeholders of clinical trials are Sponsor, Contract Research Organization (CRO), Investigator, Ethics Committee, Regulatory Authority, Patient/Study Subject.

- ☑ Sponsor takes responsibility for the initiation, management, and/or financing of a clinical trial.

- ☑ CRO is an organization contracted by the sponsor to perform one or more of a sponsor's trial-related duties and functions.

- ☑ Investigator is responsible for the conduct of a clinical trial at a site.

- ☑ Ethics committee is an independent body whose responsibility is to ensure the protection of the rights, safety and well being of human subjects involved in a clinical trial and to provide public assurance of the protection.

- ☑ Study subject is an individual who participates in a clinical trial.

4

Essential Clinical Trial Documents

Essential clinical trial documents individually and collectively evaluate the conduct of a trial and preserve the integrity of the data. These are essential to demonstrate the compliance of the investigator and sponsor/CRO with the standards of GCP and all applicable regulatory requirements.

4.1 Protocol

Document that states the background, objectives, rationale, design, methodology, (including the methods for dealing with adverse events, withdrawals *etc.*) and statistical considerations of the study.

4.2 Informed Consent Form (ICF)

A document for voluntary written consent of a subject's willingness to participate in a clinical trial that describes the rights of the study participants, and includes details about the study, such as its purpose, duration, required procedures, risks and potential benefits and key contacts.

4.3 Investigator's Brochure (IB)

Document containing data (including justification for the proposed study) for the investigator consisting of all the clinical as well as non-clinical information available on the investigational product known prior to the onset of the trial.

4.4 Case Report Form (CRF)

A printed, optical, or electronic performa designed to record all of the protocol-required information on each trial subject.

4.5 Curriculum Vitae (CV)

Document containing the details on the qualification, experience and personal information of investigator(s), sub-investigator(s), co-investigator(s), co-ordinator(s), nurse/pharmacist, sponsor designee(s) and other relevant study personnel.

4.6 Undertaking by the Investigator

A formal written, binding commitment submitted to regulatory authorities by trial investigator(s) assuring their compliance with the study protocol and all the applicable regulatory requirements.

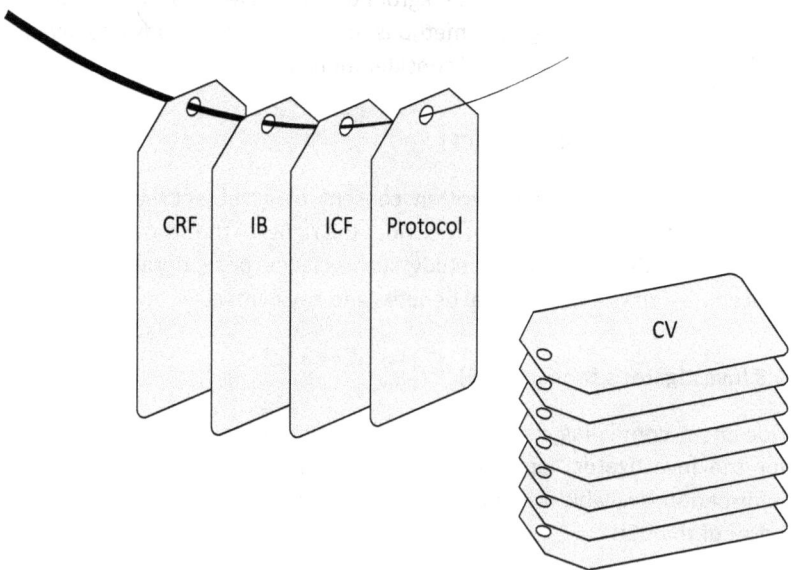

Figure 7. Essential Clinical Trial Documents

4.7 Advertisement

A document used for subject recruitment that contains non-coercive trial information and is approved by the Institutional Ethics Committee.

4.8 Clinical Trial Agreement (CTA)

A document signed and dated by the investigator and the sponsor of a trial that describes the responsibility, timelines, payment schedule and other relevant terms of agreement between the involved parties.

4.9 Insurance Statement

A legal statement that compensation for injuries related to trial drug or procedure will be available, where required.

4.10 Patient Diaries

A document given to the study subjects for recording certain observations/ readings on the condition of their health either at home or at the trial site.

4.11 Source Data

All information in original records and certified copies of original records of clinical findings, observations, or other activities in a clinical trial necessary for the reconstruction and evaluation of the trial. Source data are contained in source documents.

4.12 Source Documents

Original documents, data, and records (*e.g.*, hospital records, clinical and office charts, laboratory notes, memoranda, subject's diaries or evaluation checklists, pharmacy dispensing records, recorded data from automated instruments, copies or transcriptions certified after verification as being accurate copies, microfiches, photographic negatives, microfilm or magnetic media, x-rays, subject files, and records kept at the pharmacy, at the laboratories and at medico-technical departments involved in the clinical trial).

4.13 Certificate of Analysis

Document to provide identity, purity and strength of investigational product (s) used in a trial.

4.14 Certification/Accreditation

Evaluation of policies, working procedures and performance of an organization by an authorized body (accrediting body) to ensure that it is meeting standards laid down by accrediting body.

4.15 Clinical Study Report

Written description of the outcome of a trial enumerating the clinical and statistical interpretations.

4.16 Correspondence

Documentation of trial specific communication between various involved parties (sponsor, investigator, ERB, regulatory agency *etc.*).

4.17 Debarment List

A list published on US-FDA's website containing the names of personnel that have been disqualified for conducting clinical trials on grounds of serious misconduct or medical fraud.

4.18 Deviation File Note

A document that describes a deviation along with root cause and rectification analysis. Deviation file note contains the signature of the personnel who is responsible for the deviation and the personnel who is authorizing that deviation.

4.19 Dossier/Regulatory Dossier

A document submitted to the regulatory agencies in a pre-specified format for obtaining trial permission.

4.20 Ethics Committee Approval

Document to grant permission for the conduct of a trial at respective investigator site.

4.21 Form FDA 1572

A list of commitments and requirements by the FDA for each investigator performing drug/biologics studies.

4.22 Investigator Master File

A file that contains all the essential trial documents at a trial site.

4.23 Investigator Site Assessment Report

Refers to the detailed report prepared after reviewing the investigator's qualification, site's facility, documentation practices, storage and archival system *etc.* that forms the basis of investigator selection.

4.24 Lab Reference Range

Document containing normal values and/or ranges of the laboratory tests at the individual trial site/laboratory.

4.25 Non Disclosure Agreement (NDA)

A document that establishes agreement between two or more parties, for ensuring the confidentiality of information provided by one party to the other.

4.26 Protocol Signature Page

A document that acknowledges the investigator and/or sponsor agreement to the protocol.

4.27 Regulatory Approval

Document to grant permission for the conduct of a trial in a country.

4.28 Standard Operating Procedures (SOPs)

Detailed, written instructions to achieve uniformity of the performance of a specific function.

Summary Points

☑ Essential clinical trial documents individually and collectively evaluates the conduct of a trial and preserve the integrity of the data.

☑ These are critical to demonstrate the compliance of the investigator and sponsor/CRO with the standards of GCP and all applicable regulatory requirements.

5

Getting Started for becoming a Clinical Trial Investigator

For becoming a clinical trial investigator, a clinician is required to assume the role of a researcher in addition to his role of a clinician. There are some key differences between the routine medical care and clinical trials and it is essential to know them beforehand so that there is no conflict of interest at a later stage.

Clinical Trials	Routine Medical Care
Governed by a well-defined protocol and no changes in the therapy can be made outside the protocol specifications	Governed by the recommended standard of care and therapy can be customized based on individual patient's requirements
Follows strict inclusion-exclusion criteria	No inclusion-exclusion criteria
Requires personal involvement and commitment of the investigator in data collection, authentication and reporting	Personal involvement may or may not be present
Requires a complete follow-up and documentation of patient's medical condition, care, adverse events *etc.*	Requires very minimal follow-up and documentation of patient's medical condition, care, adverse events *etc.*
Serious Adverse Events are required to be notified to Ethics Committee	Serious Adverse Events are not required to be notified to Ethics Committee
Deadline driven and extremely time-consuming	No specific deadlines
Operates on 'science' mode	Operates on 'service' mode

Table 1. Key Difference Between Clinical Trials and Routine Medical Care

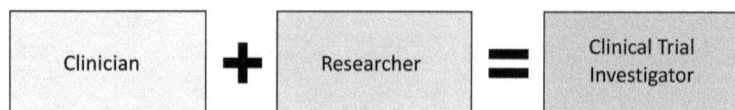

Figure 8. Becoming A Clinical Trial Investigator

Once a clinician is sure of assuming the investigator's responsibilities, the next step is to organize the essential elements required for a clinical trial investigator/site. For this a clinician is required to undertake following activities:

> Constitution of study team at the site

> Review of the composition and operating procedure of Ethics Committee

> Review and organization of the source documentation (hospital files) practices

> Review and organization of the infrastructural requirements

> Review of administrative policies and contractual obligations

Next few chapters present a detailed overview on each of the above line items.

Clinical trials can be broadly classified in two types:

> Registration studies

> Non-registration studies

5.1 Registration Studies

These studies are aimed at seeking marketing permission for potential new drug substances or for new indications (line extension) of the existing drugs. These include clinical pharmacology studies (PK/PD, drug interaction *etc.*), safety and efficacy studies (Phase-I, II, III) and line extension studies.

5.2 Non-registration Studies

These studies are aimed at gaining new information on existing drugs either in the approved indication (in-label) or a new indication (out-of-label) with the objective of using the information for planning registration studies as and when required. These include clinical trials not for registrations (CTNRs) and investigator initiated trials (IITs).

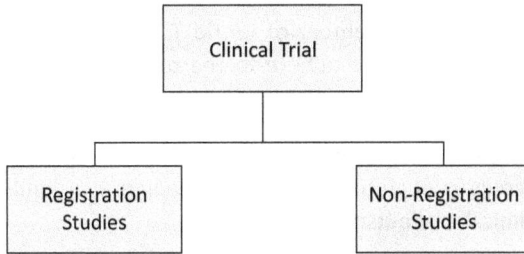

```
                    ┌─────────────────┐
                    │  Clinical Trial │
                    └─────────────────┘
                             │
            ┌────────────────┴────────────────┐
    ┌───────────────┐                 ┌───────────────────┐
    │  Registration │                 │  Non-Registration │
    │    Studies    │                 │      Studies      │
    └───────────────┘                 └───────────────────┘
```

Figure 9. Types of Clinical Trials

Advantage India

India is a nation of more than 1200 million people and second largest population in the world. India became a member of World Trade Organization (WTO) in 1995 and agreed to adhere to the product patent regime from 2005. As part of WTO, pharmaceutical industry has the rights to patent products as well as processes throughout the world including India. In the present Intellectual Property Rights (IPR) regimen, patent for a drug is valid for 20 years out of which a significant amount of time (10-12 years) is spent in development phase which is posing a big challenge to the researchers worldwide.

India clearly provides an advantage in terms of availability of large patient populations, highly skilled manpower, English speaking doctors, wide spectrum of disease, lower cost of operations, and favorable economic and IPR environment *etc.* The overall time and cost advantage in bringing a drug to the market by leveraging India could be as high as US$ 200 million. This is evident by steadily increasing number of global clinical trials in India over

29

past few years. It is estimated that more than 4500 clinical trials are being conducted in India across 5000+ investigator sites.

Summary Points

- ☑ Clinical trials are different from the routine medical care.

- ☑ India became a member of World Trade Organization (WTO) in 1995 and agreed to adhere to the product patent regime from 2005.

- ☑ India provides an advantage on the cost, speed and quality parameters of global clinical trials leading to a significant growth in clinical trial outsourcing to India.

6

Constitution of Study Team at a Trial Site

Conduct of a clinical trial requires a team effort along with the delegation of specific duties. Before participating in a clinical trial it is important for the investigator to evaluate the availability of team members.

The various personnel that constitute the study team at a trial site include:

6.1 Investigator

Investigator is a person who assumes the overall responsibility for the conduct of a clinical trial at the site. An investigator is required to have the qualification and medical license to practice a particular therapeutic area.

6.2 Co-Investigator/Sub-investigator

Co-investigator is an individual member of the clinical trial team designated and supervised by the investigator to perform critical trial-related procedures and/or to make important trial-related decisions. Co-investigator is required mainly to share investigator's responsibilities as well as to act as a back-up person when the investigator is not available. If deemed appropriate by the investigator more than one co-investigator/sub-investigator can be included in the study team.

6.3 Clinical Research Coordinator/Study Coordinator

Clinical research coordinator is a person employed at investigator's site to coordinate overall trial conduct and record the data in compliance with protocol, GCP and applicable regulatory guidelines. A dedicated study coordinator is must for the smooth execution of a clinical trial.

6.4 Research Nurse/Pharmacist

Research nurse/pharmacist is the qualified nurse/pharmacist who assists the investigator in the conduct of clinical trial. However, it is not mandatory to have them as a part of study team. Unless there is a specific requirement of involving them in the study team, their function can be delegated to the study coordinator.

6.5 Unblinded Personnel (for blinded trials only)

Unblinded personnel (study coordinator/nurse/pharmacist) are required only in blinded trials where the main study team is kept unaware of the treatment assignment. In such trials their role is to dispense the trial medication to the study subjects and act as a reference point for trial medication related emergencies.

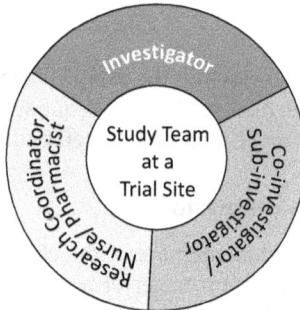

Figure 10. Composition of Study Team at a Trial Site

The composition of study team at a trial site can be a mix of above personnel. However, participation of investigator, co-investigator and study coordinator is mandatory for the smooth execution of the trial at a site. It is not mandatory to recruit all the personnel before initiating a trial as this will involve unnecessary salary expenses. But it is advisable for the investigator to have the names of potential personnel in his mind so that the same can be appointed immediately as and when required. The individual member of the study team can be delegated specific trial duties such as:

> Administration of informed consent form

- ➢ Recruitment/randomization of study subjects
- ➢ Correspondence with the Ethics Committee and Sponsor/CRO
- ➢ Storage, accountability and dispensing of investigational product
- ➢ Completion of source documents
- ➢ Completion of case report form
- ➢ Medical management of the trial subject
- ➢ Reporting of serious adverse events
- ➢ Escalation, resolution and management of deviations/violations
- ➢ Logistics management
- ➢ Resolution of data queries
- ➢ Patient's visit scheduling, follow-up and protocol compliance
- ➢ Maintenance of site master file
- ➢ Compliance with protocol, GCP and applicable regulatory guidelines
- ➢ Tracking of payments/study grants *etc.*

Constitution of study team is the first step for becoming a clinical trial investigator and once this is achieved the next steps can be undertaken.

Summary Points

☑ Study team at a clinical trial site include investigator, co-investigator, study coordinator/nurse/pharmacist.

☑ Unblinded personnel (study coordinator/nurse/pharmacist) are required in blinded trials for dispensing the trial medication to the study subjects.

☑ Clear delegation of duties to the study team members is essential for the smooth execution of a clinical trial.

7

Review of the Composition and Operating Procedure of Ethics Committee

Ethics Committee (EC) is an independent body constituted of medical/ scientific professionals and non-medical/nonscientific members, whose responsibility is to ensure the protection of rights, safety and well being of human subjects involved in a trial.

EC ensures a competent review of scientific and ethical aspects of the project proposals received and executes the same free from any bias and influence that could affect their objectivity. It might have different names at different institutions but the prime responsibility remains the same.

EC is also known as:

> ➢ Independent Ethics Committee (IEC)
> ➢ Institutional Review Board (IRB)
> ➢ Ethics Review Board (ERB)

According to Indian guidelines, EC is required to have at least 7 members with following representation:

> ➢ Basic medical scientists (preferably one pharmacologist)
> ➢ Clinicians
> ➢ Legal expert
> ➢ Social scientist / representative of non-governmental organization / philosopher /ethicist / theologian or similar person
> ➢ Lay person from the community.

Presence of at least one member each of the above representation ('quorum') is must at every EC meeting in order to qualify it as a valid meeting. The chief responsibilities of EC are:

➢ Providing its decision (*e.g.* approval/conditional approval/disapproval/ modification before approval/discontinuation of previously approved project) on the project proposals reviewed by it.

➢ Ongoing review of the progress of a clinical trial approved by it.

➢ Compliance with the regulatory requirements.

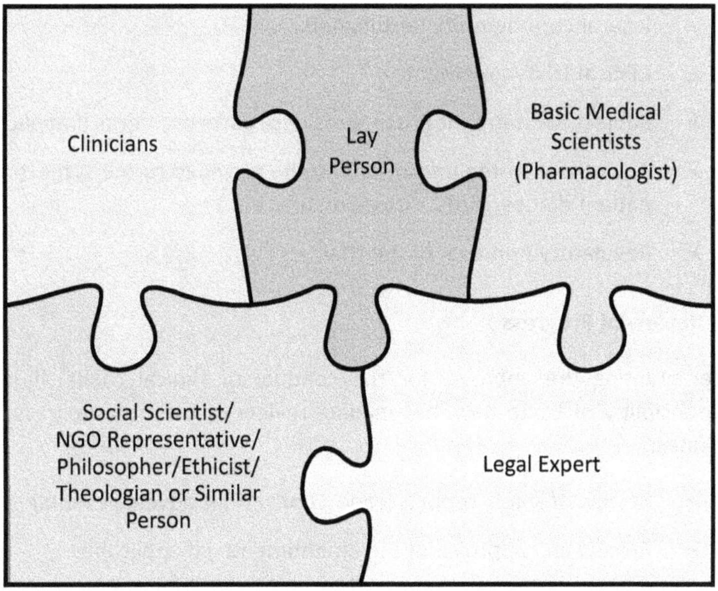

Figure 11. Composition of Ethics Committee

7.1 Approval/Permission for the Conduct of Clinical Trials

No clinical trial should be initiated at any investigator site without obtaining a written approval/permission of the essential trial documents from the respective EC. An Independent Ethics Committee can be approached if the investigator site does not have an EC of its own. Following documents requires EC review and approval before initiating a clinical trial at a site:

- ➢ Study Protocol
- ➢ Patient Information Sheet (PIS) and Informed Consent Form (ICF)
- ➢ Translations of PIS and ICF in vernacular languages along with the translation validation certificates
- ➢ Investigator's Brochure (IB) for all relevant clinical and non-clinical data on investigational product
- ➢ Undertaking by the Investigator along with recent Curriculum Vitae
- ➢ Insurance/Indemnity Certificate(s)
- ➢ Clinical Trial Agreement
- ➢ Subject Recruitment Procedures (*e.g.* advertisements if applicable)
- ➢ Any other written information to be provided to the subjects (*e.g.* patient diaries/cards, questionnaires *etc.*)
- ➢ Regulatory Approval of the trial

7.2 Review of Progress

After granting the approval for the conduct of clinical trial(s) it is the responsibility of EC to have an ongoing review of the trial progress. This includes:

- ➢ Review of safety reports (reports of serious adverse events)
- ➢ Review and approval of the amendment(s) if applicable
- ➢ Review of protocol/process deviations or violations

The frequency of these reviews may vary across institutions however it should be clearly stated in the working procedure or Standard Operating Procedure (SOP) of the EC.

7.3 Compliance with the Regulatory Requirements

In order to ensure regulatory compliance each EC is required to maintain following records:

> ➤ Written standard operating procedures or charter

> ➤ Constitution and composition as stipulated in the guidelines

> ➤ Curriculum vitae of all EC members

> ➤ Copies of all the trial(s) documents received for review

> ➤ All the correspondence between EC and investigator

> ➤ Agenda and minutes of all EC meetings

> ➤ Final report of the study

The review should be done through formal meetings and should not resort to decisions through circulation of proposals.

While ICH-GCP guidelines on the responsibilities, composition, functions and operations of EC are being practiced globally, in India far stringent norms are being recommended and followed by the ECs. Table-2 summarizes the comparison of the two guidelines.

Though the overall responsibility of the EC remains the same, Indian regulatory guidelines requires the presence of at least seven members with appropriate gender representation and chairperson from outside of the institution as compared to five members recommended by the ICH-GCP guidelines. Unlike ICH-GCP guidelines the 'quorum requirement' mentions the presence of basic medical scientist (preferably pharmacologist), legal expert and social scientist/ philosopher/ethicist/theologian or similar person also in addition to the clinicians and lay person from the community. ICH-GCP guidelines prescribe at least one continuing review per year while the Indian regulatory guideline does not specify any timelines for it.

Additionally Indian regulations require the reporting of serious and unexpected adverse events to IRB/IEC within 24 hours of their occurrence. The record retention time frame also varies between the two guidelines. Further, Indian regulation mandates the registration of Ethics Committee as per the requirements of Rule 122 DD of Drugs and Cosmetics (Third Amendment) Rules, 2013.

EC Element	ICH-GCP Guidelines[1]	Schedule-Y of Drugs & Cosmetics Act[2]
Composition and 'Quorum Requirement'	i. At least five members. ii. At least one member whose primary area of interest is in non-scientific area. iii. At least one member who is independent of the institutional/trial site. An EC may invite non-members with expertise in special area for assistance.	i. At least seven members. ii. A chairperson (who is from outside the institution) and a member secretary. iii. Other members with a mix of the medical/non-medical, scientific and non-scientific persons, including lay public, to reflect the different view points. Besides, there should be appropriate gender representation on the EC. If required, subject experts may be invited to offer their views.
Written Standard Operating Procedure	Required	Required
EC Member's list with CV	Required	Required
Review Process	EC should conduct continuing review of each ongoing trial at intervals appropriate to the degree of risk to the human subjects, but **at least once per year**. Decision should be made at announced meetings at which at least a 'quorum' as stipulated in the written operating procedures is present.	EC should make at appropriate intervals an ongoing review of the trials for which they review the protocol(s). Such a review may be based on the periodic study progress reports furnished by the investigators and/or monitoring and internal audit reports furnished by the sponsor and/or by visiting the study sites.
Voting Rights	Only those EC members who are independent of the investigator and the sponsor of the trial should vote/provide opinion on a trial related matter. Only those members who participate in the EC meeting should vote/provide their opinion and/or advise.	Only those EC members who are independent of the clinical trial and the sponsor of the trial should vote/provide opinion in matters related to study.

Safety Reporting	Investigator(s) should comply with the applicable regulatory requirements(s) related to the reporting of unexpected serious adverse drug reactions to the EC.	Investigator(s) shall report all serious and unexpected adverse events to the EC **within 24 hours** of their occurrence.
Record Keeping	The EC should retain all the relevant records for a period of at least **3 years** after the completion of the trial and make them available upon request from the regulatory authority (ies).	No mention of timelines. However, according to Indian GCP guidelines[3], all records must be safely maintained after the completion/termination of the study for at least **5 years** if it is not possible to maintain the same permanent.

Table 2. Review of ICH-GCP *vis-a-vis* Indian Regulatory Requirements on EC

The Kefauver-Harris amendments to the Federal Food and Drugs Act in 1962 increased FDA's regulatory authority over the clinical testing of new drugs. FDA periodically inspects each EC that reviews research of FDA regulated products. These inspections are either surveillance or directed.

Between January 1966 and June 2008, approximately 78 warning letters have been issued to different ECs for non-compliance[4]. Majority of violations on these warning letters includes deficiencies in review process (initial and continuing review), SOPs, quorum requirements, poor documentation, failure to report conflict of interest and protect patient's rights *etc.*

In this era of evidence based medicine when a large number of clinical trials are underway, an efficient functioning and vigilance of EC is mandatory to protect the rights and safety of the study participants. Hence, it is recommended that a potential new investigator reviews the charter/ standard operating procedures of ECs in order to ensure compliance and avoid the issuance of warning letters that can jeopardize the outcome of a clinical trial.

Summary Points

☑ EC should have written SOP on it composition, functions and operations.

☑ The composition of EC should include at least 7 members.

☑ The chairperson of EC should be from outside of the institution (non-affiliated member).

☑ The 'quorum' of EC should include at least 5 members (basic medical scientist/pharmacologist, clinician, legal expert, social scientist/ ethicist/theologian, lay person).

☑ No clinical trial should be initiated at any investigator site without obtaining a written approval from the respective EC.

☑ Version number of all the essential trial documents approved by EC should be clearly mentioned on the approval letter.

☑ All serious and unexpected adverse events should be reported to EC within 24 hours of their occurrence.

☑ If investigator or any other study team member is a part of EC, they should abstain from voting on their research proposal.

☑ EC should maintain its records for at least 5 years after the completion/termination of the study.

References:

1. http://www.ich.org [homepage on the Internet]: E6 (R1): Switzerland: Good Clinical Practice: Consolidated Guidelines. Available from: http://www.ich.org/LOB/media/MEDIA482.pdf

2. Schedule Y (Amended Version 2005). Available from: http://www.cdsco.nic.in/html/GCP1.html

3. Good Clinical Practices For Clinical Research In India. Available from: http://www.cdsco.nic.in/html/GCP1.html

4. http://www.fda.gov/[homepage on the Internet]: FDA's Electronic Freedom of Information Reading Room - Warning Letters and Responses. Available from: http://ww.fda.gov/foi/warning.htm

8

Review and Organization of the Source Documentation Practices

Clinical trial is aimed at generating valuable safety and efficacy data on an investigational product. Hence, it is imperative to have a good documentation in place that can ensure the accuracy, integrity and completeness of data. As the safety and efficacy data resides in the hospital files/OPD cards, it is important to maintain the same in such a fashion that it is readily retrievable as and when required. Also it should be able to address 'who did what' and 'when was it done' for the purpose of generating an audit trail. In clinical trials, hospital data and files are termed as source data and source document respectively.

According to ICH-GCP Guidelines, definition of source data and source document is as follows:

Source Data

All Information in original records and certified copies of original records of clinical findings, observations, or other activities in a clinical trial necessary for the reconstruction and evaluation of the trial. Source Data are contained in source documents (original records or certified copies).

Source Documents

Original documents, data, and records (*e.g.*, hospital records, clinical and office charts, laboratory notes, memoranda, subject's diaries or evaluation checklists, pharmacy dispensing records, recorded data from automated instruments, copies or transcriptions certified after verification as being accurate and complete, microfiches, photographic negatives, microfilms or magnetic media, x-rays, subject's files, and records kept at the pharmacy, at the laboratories, and at medico-technical departments involved in the clinical trial).

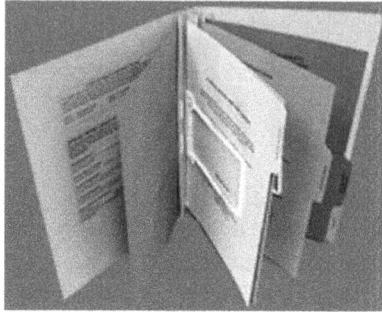

Figure 12. Source Documents

8.1 Importance of Source Data/Documents in Clinical Trials:

> Required for generating and publishing good quality data.

> Required for complete reconstruction of study during audits/ inspections.

> Required for ensuring GCP compliance and audit readiness at any given time point.

A Source Document should be maintained as per the institutional practices and should not be modified for trial purposes. However, it may contain additional information as required by the protocol. It should be stored under access control and proper environmental conditions (protection from fire, flood, termite *etc.*).

8.2 A Good Source Document includes details on:

> Patient's current medical condition and relevant history

> Laboratory reports and results

➢ Treatment administered

➢ Ongoing patient's status and notes

➢ Adverse events and corrective medications

➢ Relevant records (such as discharge summary, other treatment if any)

All the information of a patient (clinical notes, lab reports, discharge summaries, ECG tracings, radiology reports *etc.*) should be kept together in one file duly signed and dated by the concerned personnel and preferably in chronological order for the ease of navigation. If a patient is referred to another department/hospital, all the relevant records should be included in the Source Document. Source Documents should be archived for appropriate duration of time as per the institutional policies. If a clinical trial requires the Source Document to be archived for a longer duration of time, provisions should be made accordingly.

If electronic media is used for creating and storing source data instead of paper records, proper care should be taken for ensuring the security, validation and back up control mechanism.

8.3 Electronic Records as Source Documents

In August 1997, FDA's 21 CFR Part 11 regulations became effective. This regulation describes the technical and procedural requirements that must be met if electronic records and/or electronic signatures are used in lieu of paper records and signatures.

When original observations are entered directly into a computerized system, the electronic record is the source document. At some sites, source data may be held on 2 different source documents, one on paper and one as an electronic file (*e.g.* the CT Scan is held as a digital file and the report is held on paper). It is important to treat both paper and electronic files as source documents.

➢ The design of a computerized system should ensure that all applicable regulatory requirements for record keeping and record retention in clinical trials are met with the same degree of confidence as is provided with paper system.

- Validation of computerized systems should be performed to ensure accuracy, reliability and consistent performance.

- It should be documented which software, and if known, which hardware is used for electronic source data.

- In addition to internal safeguards built into the system, external safeguards should be in place to ensure that access to the computerized system and to the data is restricted to authorized personnel only (security).

- Any changes to data that are stored on electronic media should not obscure the original information. The record should clearly indicate that a change was made and clearly provide a means to locate and read the prior information (audit trail).

- Electronic source data should be retained to enable a reconstruction and evaluation of trial. The investigator/institution should take measures to prevent accidental or premature destruction of these documents (retention and archiving).

- Standard Operating Procedures pertinent to the use of the computerized systems should be available at the site (SOPs).

- Authorized site staff should be trained on the use of the system. This training should be documented (training).

A potential new investigator is advised to review the Source Documentation practices at his institute and organize them in line with the write-up above to make them acceptable to the clinical trials Sponsors/CROs.

Summary Points

☑ Source data/document constitutes the document where the information on patient's medical condition and treatment is captured for the first time.

☑ Source Document should contains accurate, authentic and complete information on patient's medical condition, laboratory results, treatment administered, adverse events and corrective medication.

☑ Proper access control should exist for the Source Document, which should be able to address 'who did what' and 'when was it done'.

☑ All the information of a patient (clinical notes, lab reports, discharge summaries, ECG tracings, radiology reports *etc.*) should be kept in one file, duly signed and dated by the concerned personnel.

☑ Source Documents should be archived for appropriate duration of time and environmental conditions.

☑ If electronic media is used for creating and storing source data instead of paper records, proper care should be taken for ensuring the security, validation and back up control mechanism.

9

Review and Organization of the Infrastructural Requirements

Conduct of clinical trials requires the presence of certain basic infrastructure at a trial site. Representative of Sponsor/CRO reviews the site infrastructure at the time of site qualification/evaluation visit and it plays an important role in getting a site selected for a clinical trial.

The basic infrastructure that is required at a trial site includes:

- ➢ Space for storing trial documents and material
- ➢ Communication facility (phone with STD/ISD facility, fax, internet *etc.*)
- ➢ Local laboratory facility
- ➢ Radiological facility (if required)
- ➢ Wards/ICUs/Operation Theatres
- ➢ Archival facility
- ➢ Standard Operating Procedures

9.1 Space for Storing Trial Document and Materials

A potential new investigator is required to have some space dedicated for conducting clinical trial. This space is required for:

- ➢ Storing trial documents (CRFs, site files, IB, source documents, training binders *etc.*)
- ➢ Storing trial material (Investigational product/comparator, lab kits, biological specimen, packaging material *etc.*)

46

> Organizing patient interviews, administration of informed consent and follow-up visits of the patients

> Execution of clinical trial activities by the study team member at the site

> Conduct of clinical trial monitoring by the Sponsor/CRO representative

This space should be equipped with:

> Lockable storage cabinets/cub-boards

> Appropriate storage facilities for storing investigational product/ comparator (*e.g.* fridge if storage temperature is 2-8°C, incubator if storage temperature is 15-25°C *etc.*)

> Deep refrigerator for storing biological specimens (if required by the trial)

> Access and environmental control (protection from fire, flood, termite *etc.*)

> Phone, fax, internet and computer access

> Power back-up

It is not necessary to have all the facilities beforehand as most of the line items mentioned above are generally procured from the trial grants. However, there should be a provision to have each one of them as and when required.

9.2 Communication Facility

A clinical trial site is required to have very good communication facilities (*e.g.* phone with STD/ISD facility, fax, internet *etc.*) in place.

Communication facilities are required for:

> Randomization of patients (either phone randomization or web randomization)

> Transmission of trial data (*e.g.* ECG tracings, data clarification form, serious adverse event reports *etc.*)

> Routine communication with Sponsor/CRO personnel as well as study subjects *etc.*

It is essential to have a direct phone line in place and the other facilities (STD/ISD, fax) can be procured from the trial grants.

9.3 Local Laboratory/Radiological Facility

Safety and efficacy assessment are the primary objective of any clinical trial and for this a potential new investigator site should be equipped with a good laboratory as well as radiological facility. However, if a site does not have these facilities it can tie-up with a service provider who is located near to the site. The laboratories should be either accredited by a National/International accreditation agency or follow the quality control standards laid down for them. Also there should be a proper access control and back-up mechanism to retrieve data of trial subjects.

In majority of trials a central laboratory is used for the purpose of achieving consistency across sites but the local laboratories are still required for managing routine medical care of the trial subjects. It is important for a potential new investigator site to procure:

> Accreditation certificate(s) of the laboratories

> Curriculum vitae(s) of the respective laboratory head

> Laboratory reference ranges

> General specification of the instruments as well as list of investigations

9.4 Wards/ICUs/Operation Theatres

These are the standard requirements for providing the medical management as well as handling the medical emergencies. However, the requirements may vary across trials and if a trial is designed to operate on OPD basis above facilities are not required.

9.5 Archival Facility

Since clinical trial documents are required to be retained for a period of 15-20 years, a potential site should be equipped with good archival facility.

Archival facility is required for:

➤ Storing the trial documents for a specified duration after the completion of a trial

➤ Preserving the trial documents for regulatory inspection/audits

➤ Ensuring compliance with applicable regulatory requirements

9.6 Standard Operating Procedures (SOPs)

Schedule-Y of Drugs and Cosmetics Act, requires every investigator site to have documented Standard Operating Procedures for the task performed by them. SOPs are detailed, written instructions to achieve uniformity in the performance of a specific function.

Typical SOPs for an investigator site should include following topics:

➤ Preparation, review and approval of SOPs

➤ Constitution of study team

➤ Feasibility assessment

➤ Ethics Committee Submission

➤ Study initiation, execution and completion

➤ Delegation of duties

➤ Administration of Informed Consent Form

➤ Reporting of Serious Adverse Event(s)

➤ Management of investigational product

➤ Record retention, update and retrieval

➤ Communication flow between team members

➤ Archival *etc.*

Following steps should be followed for creating effective SOPs:

- ➢ List down all the activities involved in the execution of a task
- ➢ List down personnel involved at each stage
- ➢ List down the delegation of specific duties
- ➢ Draw a flow chart
- ➢ Break down activities in to process stages and assign specific duties
- ➢ Review the regulatory requirements and ensure compliance
- ➢ Arrange the steps in a sequence

A potential new investigator is advised to review the available infrastructure at his institute and organize it in such a fashion that it is acceptable to the clinical trials Sponsors/CROs.

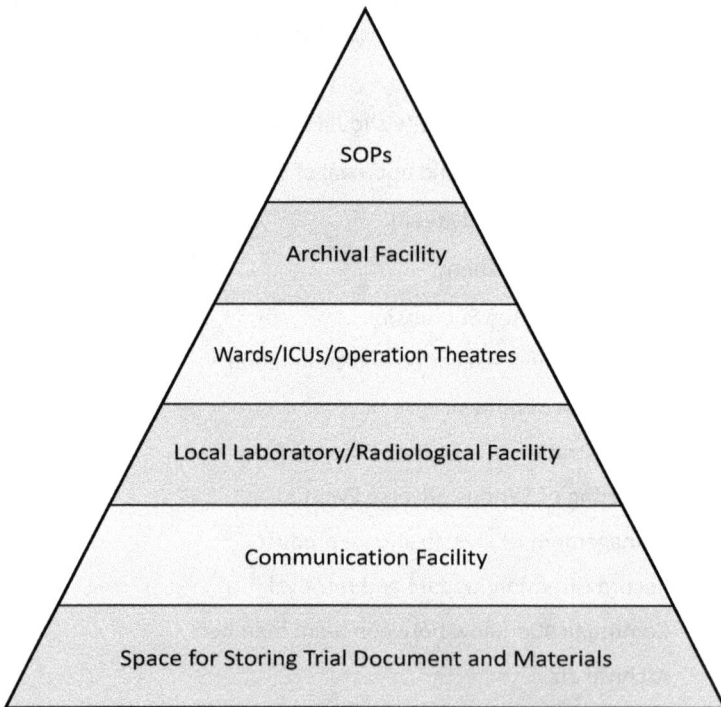

Figure 13. Review and Organization of the Infrastructural Requirements

Summary Points

☑ The basic infrastructure that is required at a trial site includes: space for storing trial documents and material, communication facility, local laboratory facility, radiological facility (if required), wards/ICUs/ operation theatres, archival facility, standard operating procedures.

☑ Trial room should be equipped with lockable storage cabinets/ cub-boards, fridge and communication facility.

☑ The laboratories to be used in a clinical trial should be either accredited by a National/International accreditation agency or follow the quality control standards laid down for them.

☑ Clinical trial documents are required to be retained for a period of 15-20 years hence a potential site should be equipped with good archival facility.

☑ A potential clinical trial site should have documented SOPs for the task performed by them.

10

Review of Administrative Policies and Contractual Obligations

The last step in getting started to become a clinical trial investigator is to review the administrative policies and contractual obligations of the institute/site. This step is critical from the legal standpoint especially in a large hospital as well as for ensuring compliance with the rules and regulations of the institute/site.

10.1 Administrative Policies

These are well defined rules and regulations of the institute/site and include policies on accepting clinical trials, recruiting study coordinator/research staff, storage and archival *etc*.

10.2 Contractual Obligations

Contractual obligations deal with the format of clinical trial agreements with the Sponsors/CROs. The format should include obligations of each party, timelines, indemnity and payment schedule. Two formats are generally being used:

➤ Tri-partite Agreements

➤ Bi-partite Agreements

Tri-partite Agreements involves three parties namely Sponsor/CRO, Investigator and Head of the institution/designee. This is the best way of executing a clinical trial agreement and offers certain advantages.

Advantage of Tri-partite Agreements are as follows:

➤ Each of the three party bears a joint responsibility of executing the clinical trial at the site

➤ Brings transparency in the conduct of clinical trial

➤ Ensures compliance with institutional policies on accepting the study grant

➤ Obligation of the institution for storage and archival of trial documents for a specified period of time becomes extremely important if the investigator leaves the institution during this time-frame

Bi-partite Agreement on the other hand is executed between the Sponsor/ CRO and the investigator only. In this case institute does not have any obligation with regards to the conduct of clinical trial. In addition this arrangement may jeopardize the outcome of a trial whenever investigator leaves the institution.

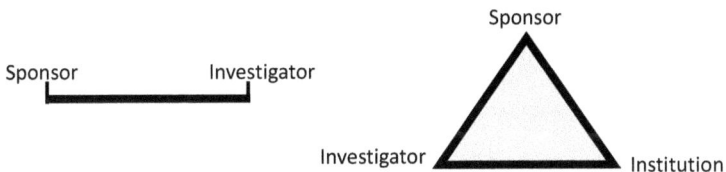

Figure 14. Bi-Partite and Tri-partite Clinical Trial Agreement

A potential new investigator is advised to review the administrative policies and contractual obligations at his institute in order to ensure compliance in the conduct of a clinical trial.

At this stage it also becomes useful to collect information on number of patients (disease-wise) registered at the institution/site over a period of time (generally over last 1 year). This information is essential to judge the enrolment potential of the site and can become a deciding factor for a Sponsor/CRO to select the site for a particular trial.

Once a potential new investigator fix-up the action items described in

Chapters 5 to 10, his site becomes ready to begin the participation in a clinical trial.

Next few Chapters provide an insight on how to initiate a clinical trial at the site.

Summary Points

☑ Administrative policies are well defined rules and regulations of the institute/site and include policies on accepting clinical trials, recruiting research staff, storage and archival *etc.*

☑ Two formats of clinical trial agreements are generally being used: Tri-partite Agreements and Bi-partite Agreements.

☑ Tri-partite Agreement is the best way of executing the clinical trial agreement as the institution's obligations of archiving the trial documents for a specified period of time becomes very important whenever the investigator leaves the institution during this time-frame.

11

Beginning the Participation in a Clinical Trial: Site Evaluation/ Qualification Visit

A potential new investigator site can begin it's participation in a clinical trial either by directly approaching the Sponsors/CROs or increasing its visibility for getting approached by the Sponsors/CROs. In both the scenarios the deciding factors for selection of a new site include:

- ➢ Investigator's qualification and experience
- ➢ Enrolment potential of the site which in turn is linked to number of patients seen by the investigator for the disease condition under study
- ➢ Investigator's commitment and willingness to spare time for the trial
- ➢ Availability of co-investigator and other team members
- ➢ Availability of an Ethics Committee having the composition and written operating procedures in compliance with the applicable regulatory requirements
- ➢ Source documentation practices of the site
- ➢ Availability of the basic infrastructure
- ➢ Administrative policies related to the execution of clinical trial agreement

Whenever a new investigator site is being approached for participation in a clinical trial the first step is execution of a Non Disclosure Agreement (NDA) between the Sponsor/CRO and the Investigator. This agreement establishes the obligation on the part of investigator for maintaining the confidentiality of information being provided to him/discussed with him by the Sponsor/ CRO designee. Once NDA is executed, Sponsor/CRO designee forwards a study feasibility questionnaire/protocol synopsis/brief study outline to the Investigator or discusses it over phone. If the response of the investigator on the study feasibility questionnaire meets the expectations of the Sponsor/ CRO, a site evaluation/qualification visit is organised at the investigator site. Based on the outcome of the visit, a new investigator site is either selected or rejected for participation in a clinical trial. However, if the site meets all the pre-requisite requirements it is highly unlikely that it gets rejected.

The **process flow** for the Site Evaluation/Selection activity is as follows:

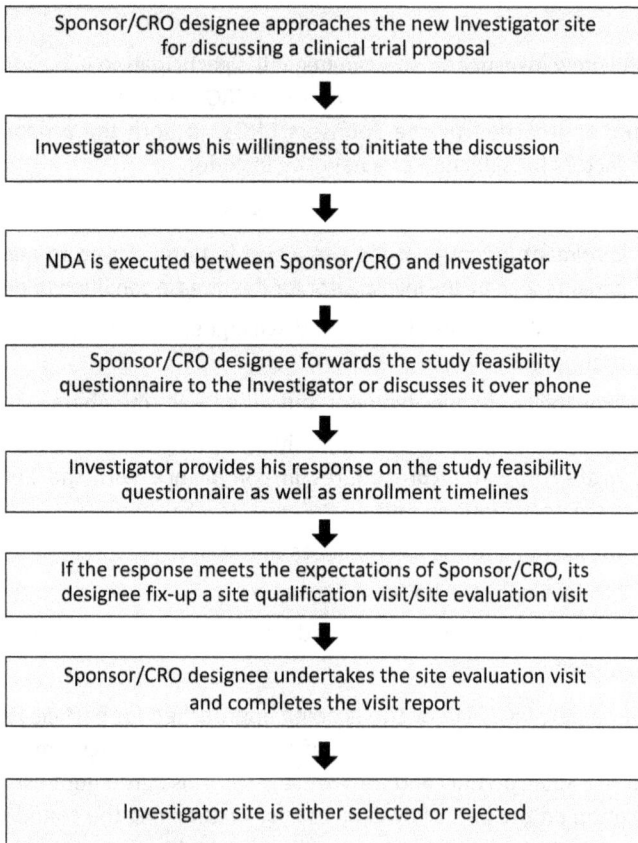

Sponsor/CRO designee approaches the new Investigator site for discussing a clinical trial proposal

⬇

Investigator shows his willingness to initiate the discussion

⬇

NDA is executed between Sponsor/CRO and Investigator

⬇

Sponsor/CRO designee forwards the study feasibility questionnaire to the Investigator or discusses it over phone

⬇

Investigator provides his response on the study feasibility questionnaire as well as enrollment timelines

⬇

If the response meets the expectations of Sponsor/CRO, its designee fix-up a site qualification visit/site evaluation visit

⬇

Sponsor/CRO designee undertakes the site evaluation visit and completes the visit report

⬇

Investigator site is either selected or rejected

Summary Points

☑ Non Disclosure Agreement establishes the obligation on the part of investigator for maintaining the confidentiality of information provided to him by the Sponsor/CRO.

☑ Sponsor/CRO designee undertakes the site evaluation visit and reviews the qualification of study team members, composition and operating procedure of EC, source documentation practices and infrastructure *etc.*

☑ Based on the outcome of the site evaluation/qualification visit, a new investigator site is either selected or rejected for participation in a clinical trial.

12

Beginning the Participation in a Clinical Trial: Site Activation

Based on the successful outcome of the site evaluation/qualification visit an investigator site is selected for participation in a clinical trial. At this stage Sponsor/CRO designee forwards the following documents to the Investigator for review and completion:

- ➢ Study Protocol

- ➢ Patient Information Sheet (PIS) and Informed Consent Form (ICF) in English

- ➢ Translation of PIS and ICF in required vernacular languages based on the geographical location of the site

- ➢ Translation and Validation Certificate

- ➢ Investigator's Brochure (IB)

- ➢ Case Report Form (CRF)

- ➢ Insurance/Indemnity Certificate

- ➢ Patient diaries/questionnaires/any other information to be provided to study subjects (if applicable)

- ➢ Format of Undertaking by the Investigator

- ➢ Draft of Clinical Trial Agreement (CTA)

- ➢ Regulatory clearance (DCGI approval) of the trial if available

Once the above documents are received at the investigator site, he is required to undertake following activity:

- Acknowledge the receipt
- Sign/date on the protocol signature page
- Sign/date on the IB receipt form
- Review ICF translations for accuracy and completeness
- Complete the details on Undertaking by the Investigator followed by printing it on the letter head for signatures
- Review the CTA for the overall study grant as well as payment schedule and execute the same

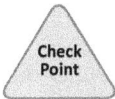

Check Point

As the payment schedule in the CTA is generally linked to achieving a particular milestone it becomes extremely important to ensure that:

- Payment schedule is linked to an optimal milestone (for *e.g.* if the CTA states that payment will be made after 5 patients are enrolled in the study than the investigator should evaluate the time frame for recruiting 5 patients as well as the scenario in which site recruits less than 5 patients and suggests the required changes accordingly)
- Payment is made for all screen failures (study subjects who fails to meet the inclusion criteria)
- Advance payment is available to take care of the payment delays
- Payment for research staff (study coordinator) is made on monthly basis rather than linking it to a milestone
- Payment for the administrative/infrastructural costs is made at the beginning of the trial
- EC fee is paid directly and not linked to the CTA

An ideal CTA is yet to be evolved and majority of time investigator site faces problem with regards to delay in receiving payment, frequent amendments in the payment schedule, retaining the dedicated study personnel without monthly payment *etc.* However, most of these issues can be avoided if the investigator reviews the CTA carefully and suggests the appropriate amendments to the Sponsor/CRO.

In addition to the above documents based on the requirement of the applicable regulatory authority; Sponsor/CRO designee obtains Statement of Investigator (*e.g.* FDA 1572), Financial Disclosure Forms, CV and Medical Registration Certificate from the investigator.

At this stage, site becomes ready to submit the essential trial documents to the respective Ethics Committee (EC) for its review and opinion. Based on the operating procedure, required number of copies of the essential documents is submitted to the EC. Once the site receives the EC approval it becomes absolutely ready to initiate the study. Sponsor/CRO sends all the initial site supplies (case report forms, investigator site file, investigational product, lab kits *etc.*) at this stage.

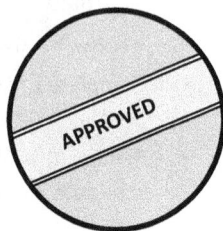

Between the time of EC submission and approval a Sponsor/CRO may undertake the training of investigator and other study team members. Generally a common investigator training meeting is organized and all the participating investigators are invited to a common location along with their team members. The objective of investigator training meeting is to provide a uniform understanding on following topics to all the participants :

➢   Good Clinical Practice guidelines

➢   Protocol and product overview

➢   ICF process

➢   Safety reporting

➢   Completion of case report form and data management

➢   Accountability and management of investigational product

➢   Investigator site file management and update

➢   Roles and responsibilities of site personnel

➢   Central lab (if applicable)

➢   Audits and inspections

➢   Study timelines *etc.*

Once the training is provided to the investigator team on study protocol/ processes and EC and regulatory approvals are in place, the next step is to initiate the site.

Summary Points

☑ Based on the successful outcome of the site qualification visit an investigator site is selected for participation in a clinical trial.

☑ Investigator forwards essential trial documents (study protocol, PIS and ICF, translations, IB, CRF, insurance/indemnity certificate, undertaking by the Investigator, CTA, regulatory clearance *etc.*) to the respective EC for its review and opinion.

☑ A careful review of the draft CTA by the investigator and subsequent suggestions (if any) can avoid issues such as payment delays, frequent amendments, retaining the dedicated study personnel without monthly payment *etc.*

☑ The objective of investigator training meeting is to provide a uniform understanding of protocol and processes to all the participants.

13

Site Initiation

Site initiation refers to the process of assessing the readiness of an investigator site for initiating the enrolment in a clinical trial. Site initiation visit is performed after the Ethics approval and prior to first patient visit (FPV) to ensure that the investigator and the site personnel are trained on various clinical trial responsibilities.

Site initiation visit is generally performed in person by the Sponsor/CRO designee (study monitor) to review and verify that the investigator and his team are trained on the clinical trial requirements, which include:

- ➢ Essential Trial Documents
- ➢ Roles and Responsibilities/Delegations
- ➢ Facility
- ➢ Informed Consent Process
- ➢ Serious Adverse Event (SAE) Process
- ➢ Ethics Committee (EC) Requirements
- ➢ Study Drug Storage and Accountability
- ➢ Source Documents
- ➢ Randomization Procedure
- ➢ Data Management
- ➢ Role of Sponsor

> ➤ Study Timelines
> ➤ Audits/Inspections
> ➤ Archival *etc.*

13.1 Essential Trial Documents

The training on essential trial documents is must in order to generate good quality scientific data. The essential trial documents include:

> ➤ Protocol
> ➤ Informed Consent Document
> ➤ Case Report Form (CRF)
> ➤ Investigator's Brochure (IB)
> ➤ Training Binder
> ➤ Investigator Master File *etc.*

The investigator and his team should be clear on the inclusion/exclusion criteria and protocol schedule of events in order to avoid violations that can jeopardize the trial results/outcome. The team should also be clear on the critical junctures in the protocol and should refer to protocol regularly in order to ensure compliance. Investigator Master File should include all the essential documents required to be present at the time of beginning the study.

13.2 Roles and Responsibilities/Delegations

It is extremely important to define 'who would do what' to ensure compliance with ICH-GCP and applicable regulatory requirements. This includes defining the roles and responsibilities of:

> ➤ Investigator
> ➤ Co-investigator(s)
> ➤ Sub-investigator(s)
> ➤ Study Coordinator(s)
> ➤ Study Nurse/Pharmacist

> Social worker/Administrative staff (if applicable)

The roles and responsibilities should be properly documented with signature of concerned person against his/her delegations. Generally a back up is kept for each role to maintain continuity.

13.3 Facility

After the investigator assessment visit the study monitor reviews the facility once again at site initiation visit to ensure that it remain adequate for conducting the proposed clinical trial. It includes review of:

> Communication facilities (telephone, fax, e-mail with STD/ISD connections)

> Study drug storage devices (refrigerator, air-conditioner)

> Deep refrigerator for storing biological samples (if required)

> Trial room/cupboards

> Laboratory and imaging facility

> Pharmacy

> Medical records section

If there is any deficiency in the facility, it should be resolved prior to initiating the patient enrolment.

13.4 Informed Consent Process

Informed consent is a process by which a subject voluntarily confirms his or her willingness to participate in a particular trial, after having been informed of all aspects of the trial that are relevant to the subject's decision to participate. Informed consent is documented by means of a written, signed and dated informed consent form. An investigator site is expected to be fully trained on informed consent process in order to protect the rights, safety and well being of trial subjects. It includes:

> Delegation for obtaining the informed consent form

➤ Steps for obtaining the informed consent from literate patients

➤ Steps for obtaining the informed consent from illiterate patients

➤ Steps for obtaining the informed consent from special population

➤ Appropriate use of translations

➤ Documentation requirements

➤ Need for providing a copy of signed informed consent to the subject

A lot of violations can be avoided by addressing the training needs of the site on informed consent process.

13.5 Serious Adverse Event (SAE) Process

Serious adverse event constitutes an important safety element of a trial. The investigator site is required to be trained on SAE process to ensure ICH-GCP and regulatory compliance. It includes training on:

➤ Definition of a valid case

➤ Adverse event management guidelines

➤ Reporting timelines

➤ Filling up of an SAE form

➤ Follow-up requirements

➤ EC notification and compliance

Any deviations in SAE reporting can lead to significant audit findings.

13.6 Ethics Committee (EC) Requirements

The investigator site is required to be trained on EC requirements and compliance, which includes:

➤ Constitution, function and operations of EC

- ➤ Written operating procedures

- ➤ Approval of protocol, informed consent form with translations, investigator brochure and other essential trial documents

- ➤ If the investigator or co-investigator is a member of the EC, their non-participation in the voting process should be documented in the approval letter

- ➤ Approval of all advertisements

- ➤ Periodic and ongoing reporting of SAE, trial progress, trial suspension or completion to EC

13.7 Study Drug Storage and Accountability

Study drug accountability is an essential regulatory requirement and the investigator sites are expected to maintain 100% drug accountability at any given moment of time. During the site initiation visit the training of investigator site is assessed on study drug accountability, which includes:

- ➤ Storage requirements of the drug

- ➤ Reconstitution guidelines (if applicable)

- ➤ Access control

- ➤ Completion of drug accountability logs

- ➤ Completion of temperature logs

- ➤ Maintenance of accountability of all used and unused drug

- ➤ Maintenance of inventory control

- ➤ Reporting of non-compliance

- ➤ Dispensing of study drug only to study subjects

13.8 Source Documents

Training on source documents includes:

- ➤ Discussion on what constitutes source document at a particular site

> ➢ Discussion on the form in which the source document is available at a particular site (for *e.g.* paper or electronic)

> ➢ Recording of trial specific information

> ➢ Investigator's or designee's review and sign-offs

> ➢ Access control

> ➢ Availability of source documents during monitoring visits

> ➢ Storage and archival of the source documents for the required duration

> ➢ Regulatory compliance for the electronic source documents

13.9 Randomization Procedure

During the site initiation visit randomization procedure is explained to the site personnel. If it requires demonstration on an Interactive Voice Response System the same is generally performed. Blinding and unblinding procedures (if applicable) are also discussed in detail.

13.10 Data Management

Data management refers to defining the paper flow process for managing the trial data. It includes training on:

> ➢ CRF completion

> ➢ Query resolution

> ➢ Co-ordination with the data management center

> ➢ Filing of queries with the respective CRF pages

13.11 Role of Sponsor

Training on the role of sponsor includes:

> ➢ Discussion on the role of monitor and other sponsor designee

> Contact information of the monitor and the designee

> Discussion on the requirements of a monitoring visit

13.12 Study Timelines

In any clinical trial, study timelines are of prime importance. Investigator site should be informed about the study timelines well in advance in order to avoid study delays. This includes discussion on:

> Projected first patient visit

> Projected last patient visit

> Enrolment rate

> Data cut-off dates

> Study closure dates

13.13 Audits/Inspections

During the site initiation visit, investigator site is trained on the requirements of audits/inspections, which include:

> Relevance and significance of audits/inspections

> Process of investigator's site audit

> Importance of compliance with ICH-GCP and the applicable local laws and regulations

> Follow-up on audit findings/report

13.14 Archival

Clinical trial record retention and archival is a regulatory requirement. Investigator site is trained on archival of trial documents, which include:

> Archival requirements and recommendations
> Archival location
> Access control *etc.*

Site initiation activities are essential to obtain the desired results in a particular trial. Most of the scientific, regulatory and logistic issues are addressed during the site initiation visit leaving behind a very little scope of deviations/violations. Moreover, it provides the investigator site an opportunity to re-visit the critical aspects of a clinical trial after the initial training and before the implementation phase. During the site initiation visit critical study supplies are also checked and if the site has all the supplies in place, it is given clearance for recruiting the study subjects.

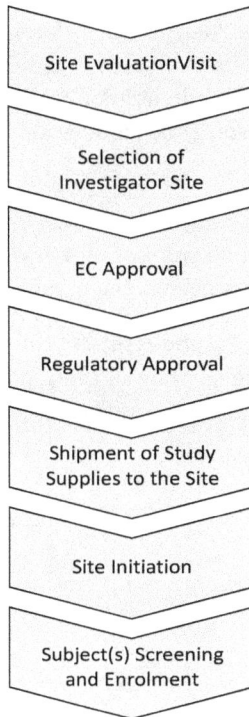

Figure 15. Stages from Site Evaluation Visit to Subject Enrolment

Summary Points

☑ Site initiation visit is performed to assess the readiness of an investigator site for initiating the enrolment in a clinical trial.

☑ Site initiation visit is performed after the Ethics approval and prior to first patient visit.

☑ Site initiation visit is performed in person by the study monitor to review and verify that the investigator and his team are trained on the clinical trial requirements: trial documents, roles and responsibilities/delegations, informed consent process, SAE process, EC requirements, study drug storage and accountability, source documents, randomization procedure, data management, role of the Sponsor/CRO, study timelines, audits/inspections, archival *etc.*

☑ Site initiation visit provides the investigator site an opportunity to re-visit the critical aspects of a clinical trial after the initial training and before the implementation phase.

☑ During the site initiation visit, critical study supplies are also checked and if the site has all the supplies in place, it is given clearance for recruiting the study subjects.

14

ICF Administration and Patient Enrolment

At this stage potential subjects (whom the investigator feels can qualify the inclusion/exclusion criteria) are screened for inclusion in the clinical trial. The first step in this process is to obtain an Informed Consent. Informed consent is a process by which a subject voluntarily confirms his or her willingness to participate in a particular trial, after having been informed of all aspects of the trial that are relevant to the subject's decision to participate. Informed consent is documented by means of a written, signed and dated Informed Consent Form (ICF).

The ICF is used to explain the risks and benefits of study participation to the subject in simple terms and vernacular language, before the subject participates in the study. ICH-GCP section 4.8.10 contains a description of 20 essential elements [section 4.8.10(a) to 4.8.10(t)] required to be included in the ICF. Similarly Indian guidelines also recommends essential element for an ICF. It is the responsibility of Sponsor to ensure that ICF contains all the relevant details and description as specified by the applicable regulatory guidelines. Additionally, Indian regulation also mandates the audio-visual recording of the informed consent process.

14.1 Requirements of obtaining Informed Consent in a Clinical Trial:

➢ The investigator, or a person knowledgeable about the trial and designated by the investigator, must obtain informed consent

➢ Informed Consent must be obtained before non-routine screening procedures are performed and/or before any change in the subject's current medical therapy is made for the purpose of the clinical trial

- ➤ The subject (or subject's legally acceptable representative) should have ample opportunity to ask questions and to decide whether or not to participate in the clinical trial

- ➤ The subject should not be coerced to participate or continue the participation in a trial

- ➤ The subject (or subject's legally acceptable representative*) and the individual obtaining consent must personally sign and date (with the time, where appropriate) the ICF

- ➤ The signature of the prospective subject or legal representative on the ICF indicates that the content of the ICF has been adequately discussed, and that the informed consent was freely given by the subject or legal representative

- ➤ The subject or legal representative should receive a copy of the signed ICF and any subsequent amendments

- ➤ In situation where the subject can be enrolled in a trial only with the consent of a legal representative, (e.g., minors, or subjects with severe dementia), the subject should be informed of the clinical trial to the level of subject's understanding. In addition to the legally acceptable representative, the subject should (if capable) personally sign and date (with time, if appropriate) the ICF

- ➤ In case of an ICF amendment study subject(s) who have already consented should re-consent on the new version of the Ethics Committee approved ICF and the same should be used for all new enrolments

14.2 Special Circumstances:

- ➤ In emergency situations, when prior consent of the subject is not possible, the consent of the subject's legally acceptable representative, if present, should be obtained

- ➤ When prior consent of the subject is not possible, and the subject's legally acceptable representative is unable to be physically present to read and sign the ICF, or a legally acceptable representative is

---

* An individual or juridical or other body authorized under applicable law to consent, on behalf of a prospective subject, to the subject's participation in the clinical trial.

not available, enrolment of the subject should require measures described in the protocol and/or elsewhere, with documented approval/favorable opinion by the Ethics Committee. The subject or the subject's legally acceptable representative should be informed about the trial as soon as possible and consent to continue should be requested

➢ In situations where the subject or subject's legally acceptable representative is unable to read, an impartial witness** should be present during the informed consent discussions. After oral consent has been obtained from the subject or subject's legally acceptable representative, and after the subject or subject's legally acceptable representative has signed and dated the ICF (if he/she is capable of doing so), the witness should also sign and date the ICF

This signature and date indicates that the information in the consent form was accurately explained to the subject or subject's legally acceptable representative and that informed consent was freely given by the subject or subject's legally acceptable representative.

14.3 Essential Elements of Data Privacy Statement:

All ICF should contained a data privacy statement to include,

➢ Description of information to be used or disclosed
➢ Specific identification of the persons authorized to make the requested use or disclosure
➢ Specific identification of the persons to whom the covered entity may make the requested use or disclosure
➢ Statement regarding purpose of use/disclosure
➢ Statement regarding explanation of Authorization
➢ Statement of the individual's right to revoke the Authorization
➢ Statement that the sponsor will not disclose personal health information to insurance companies unless required to do so by law, or unless subject(s) provides a separate written consent to do so.

** A person, who is independent of the trial, who cannot be unfairly influenced by people involved with the trial, who attends the informed consent process if the subject or the subject's legally acceptable representative cannot read, and who reads the informed consent form and any other written information supplied to the subject.

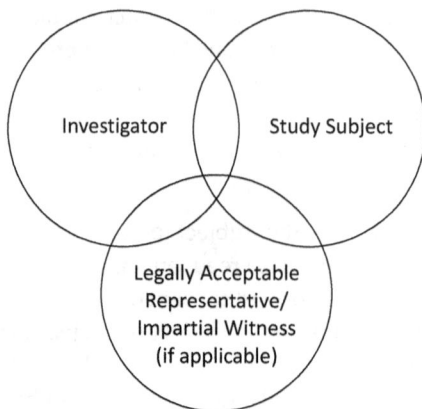

Figure 16. ICF Administration Process

14.4 Process Flow for Obtaining Informed Consent Form from Literate Subject (s):

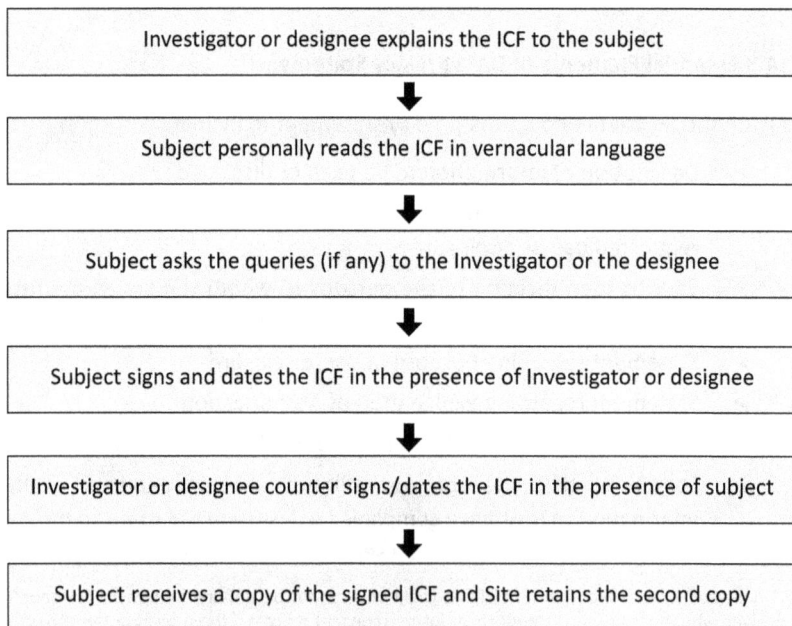

Investigator or designee explains the ICF to the subject

⬇

Subject personally reads the ICF in vernacular language

⬇

Subject asks the queries (if any) to the Investigator or the designee

⬇

Subject signs and dates the ICF in the presence of Investigator or designee

⬇

Investigator or designee counter signs/dates the ICF in the presence of subject

⬇

Subject receives a copy of the signed ICF and Site retains the second copy

14.5 Process Flow for Obtaining Informed Consent Form from Illiterate Subject(s):

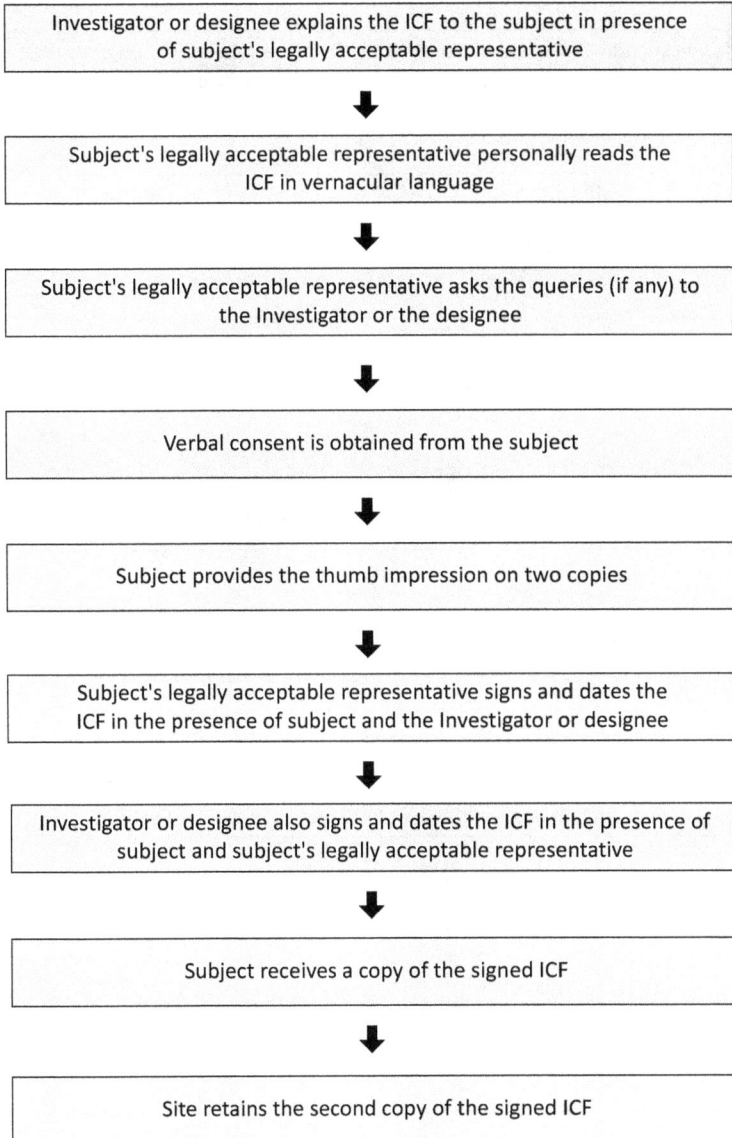

Investigator or designee explains the ICF to the subject in presence of subject's legally acceptable representative

⬇

Subject's legally acceptable representative personally reads the ICF in vernacular language

⬇

Subject's legally acceptable representative asks the queries (if any) to the Investigator or the designee

⬇

Verbal consent is obtained from the subject

⬇

Subject provides the thumb impression on two copies

⬇

Subject's legally acceptable representative signs and dates the ICF in the presence of subject and the Investigator or designee

⬇

Investigator or designee also signs and dates the ICF in the presence of subject and subject's legally acceptable representative

⬇

Subject receives a copy of the signed ICF

⬇

Site retains the second copy of the signed ICF

14.6 Process Flow for Obtaining Informed Consent Form when both Subject and Subject's Legally Acceptable Representative (LAR) are Illiterate:

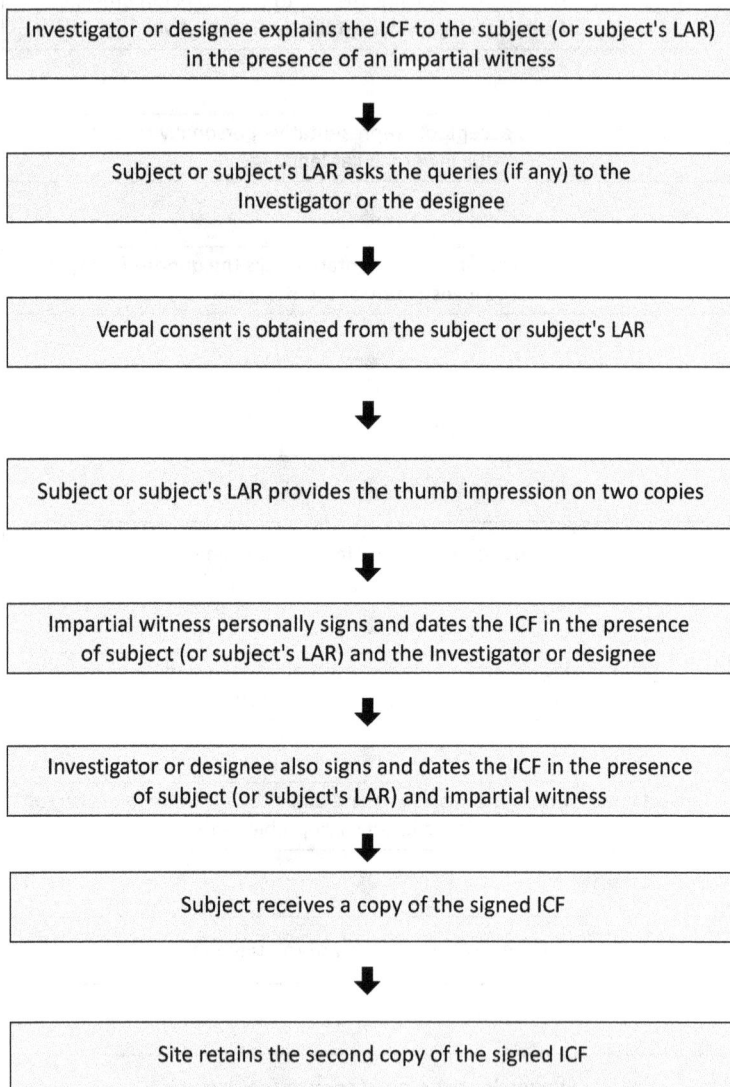

Investigator or designee explains the ICF to the subject (or subject's LAR) in the presence of an impartial witness

⬇

Subject or subject's LAR asks the queries (if any) to the Investigator or the designee

⬇

Verbal consent is obtained from the subject or subject's LAR

⬇

Subject or subject's LAR provides the thumb impression on two copies

⬇

Impartial witness personally signs and dates the ICF in the presence of subject (or subject's LAR) and the Investigator or designee

⬇

Investigator or designee also signs and dates the ICF in the presence of subject (or subject's LAR) and impartial witness

⬇

Subject receives a copy of the signed ICF

⬇

Site retains the second copy of the signed ICF

14.7 Tips on Obtaining ICF

☞ **Always make sure that**

➤ ICF contains all the elements specified by the ICH GCP and applicable regulatory requirements

➤ Subject personally reads the ICF in vernacular language

➤ Subject (or legally acceptable representative) gets the opportunity to ask the queries (if any) to the Investigator or the designee

➤ Subject receives a copy of the signed ICF

Voluntary consent is must for protecting the rights, safety and well being of subject(s)

☞ **Ensure that**

➤ A version date and a version number identifies an ICF

➤ Version control is maintained for all subsequent amendments

➤ Translation in vernacular languages is approved by EC

➤ Only the EC approved version of ICF is administered to the study subject(s)

Version control is vital to ensure GCP compliance

☞ **Make sure that**

➤ Investigator or designee personally obtains the ICF from the subject

➤ Delegation of obtaining ICF is clearly documented in the trial file

➤ ICF is obtained before non-routine screening procedures are performed and/or before any change in the subject's current medical therapy is made for the purpose of the clinical trial

ICF should be obtained only by the investigator or designee

☞ **Don't ever forget to take**

➤ Signature of the literate subject(s) on the ICF of the required vernacular language

➤ Oral consent and thumb impression of illiterate subject(s) followed by the signature of subject's legally acceptable representative

➤ Oral consent and thumb impression of illiterate subject(s) or subject's legally acceptable representative who is illiterate followed by the signature of an impartial witness

Regulatory and GCP compliance is must in any clinical trial to avoid non-compliance

☞ **Always make sure that**

➤ In case of an ICF amendment, study subject(s) who have already consented, re-consents on the new version of the document

➤ All new subject(s) signs on to the new version only

➤ Previous version(s) is marked as "invalid" or "superseded" or "do not use" and kept separately

➤ A tracking log is maintained to record version(s) control

Good practice and ethics leads to scientifically and ethically sound study

14.8 Patient Enrolment

After obtaining the ICF, screening tests are performed and subjects who qualify inclusion/exclusion criteria are enrolled in the trial. Once a subject is enrolled in a clinical trial, protocol schedule of events should be followed strictly in order to ensure 100% compliance.

An investigator site can use the following tips for ensuring protocol compliance:

➤ Protocol schedule of events should be thoroughly clear to all the members of study team

➤ A one page handout for the protocol schedule of events can be kept as a quick reference point

➢ Visit based checklist can be designed to include all the activities at a particular visit and the same can be filled every time a patient comes for a scheduled visit

➢ Study coordinator can keep a track of patient's visit and remind them of their next scheduled visit

➢ Critical junctures of the protocol (*e.g.* dose modification, discontinuation *etc.*) should always be checked as and where applicable

Data as required by the protocol should be carefully recorded in the source document at each visit and the same should be transcribed into the case report form. Appropriate medical care should be provided to the study subject throughout the trial duration.

Summary Points

☑ Informed consent is a process by which a subject voluntarily confirms his or her willingness to participate in a particular trial, after having been informed of all aspects of the trial that are relevant to the subject's decision to participate.

☑ It is the responsibility of Sponsor to ensure that ICF contains all the relevant details and description as specified by the applicable regulatory guidelines.

☑ Informed Consent must be obtained before non-routine screening procedures are performed and/or before any change in the subject's current medical therapy is made for the purpose of the clinical trial.

☑ The subject (or subject's legally acceptable representative) and the individual obtaining consent must personally sign and date (with the time, where appropriate) the ICF.

☑ One copy of the signed ICF should always be given to the subject.

☑ ICF should be obtained only by the investigator or designee.

☑ In situations where the subject or subject's legally acceptable representative is unable to read, an impartial witness should be present during the informed consent discussions.

☑ In case of an ICF amendment study subject(s) who have already consented should re-consent on the new version of the Ethics Committee approved ICF and the same should be used for all new enrolments.

☑ Data required by the protocol should be carefully recorded in the source document at each visit and the same should be transcribed into the case report form on a regular basis.

15

Maintenance of Source Document

It is the responsibility of investigator site to maintain the source document for each trial patient. Source Document should be able to tell the complete story and one should be able to reconstruct the entire trial simply on the basis of information captured in the Source Document. All the information should be accurately recorded along with an audit trail of who did what and when it was done. It is a good practice to highlight a patient's participation in a clinical trial on the cover page of the Source Document.

The use of Case Report Forms (CRFs) as Source Document should be limited only to certain parameters like Quality of Life questionnaires, Evaluation scales, Patient demographics *etc.* and it should be mentioned in the Protocol.

A good Source Document should be able to address the following:

- ➢ ICF process
- ➢ Pre-existing conditions and relevant history
- ➢ Laboratory reports and results
- ➢ Efficacy evaluations *e.g.* radiological investigations, blood glucose monitoring, patient's response *etc.*
- ➢ Adverse events and corrective medications
- ➢ Drug accountability
- ➢ Progress notes
- ➢ Patient's status (ongoing) *etc.*

15.1 ICF Process

Since voluntary consent is mandatory in any clinical trial, ICF process should always be documented. This includes a mention of:

> - Whether the patient is literate or illiterate
> - Who was the legal representative in case of illiterate patient
> - Who was the impartial witness in case of illiterate patient with no legal representative or illiterate legal representative
> - Which translation was used
> - The queries/questions that the patient/legal representative had asked

If the patient withdraws the consent during the course of a trial, it should be recorded in the source document along with the reason (if any).

15.2 Pre-existing Conditions and Relevant Medical History

All pre-existing conditions and the relevant present and past medical history including therapy undergone by the patient with duration should be included at the time of taking the initial notes. This includes a mention of:

> - Start date of pre-existing conditions
> - Severity grade of pre-existing conditions
> - Corrective medications for pre-existing conditions
> - Stop date of significant historical diagnosis

These should be followed on an ongoing basis.

15.3 Laboratory Reports and Results

The laboratory results are an important safety parameter and critical for assessing the side effects with the investigational product. All the laboratory reports and results should be maintained properly since this is a focus area during regulatory inspections.

> - All lab reports should be placed in chronological order and should be duly signed by the reporter and the investigator/designee

- ➤ All values that are out of reference range should be commented upon if they are clinically significant
- ➤ Any dosing decision related to laboratory values should be taken only after the investigator has reviewed, noted his comments and signed the lab reports
- ➤ Whitener should not be applied on the lab reports to obscure or correct any value
- ➤ Thermal printouts (from the automated machines) should be enclosed along with the lab reports for providing an audit trail

15.4 Efficacy Evaluations

Almost all of the clinical trials are geared towards ascertaining the safety and efficacy of investigational product. While safety is assessed using the laboratory results, efficacy is assessed from the relevant diagnostic evaluation or from the patient's response when diagnostic evaluation is not possible. It includes radiological investigations for oncology trials; blood glucose monitoring for diabetes trials and patient's response for psychiatry trials *etc.*

Radiological investigations

- ➤ Should be on the same format, covering the same area across visits
- ➤ All reports should be placed in chronological order and should be duly signed by the reporter and the investigator/designee
- ➤ The films should be present in original and should not be physically altered *e.g.* bent/ folded/ cut

Blood glucose monitoring

- ➤ All reports should be placed in chronological order and should be duly signed by the reporter and the investigator/designee
- ➤ Patient's response should be verifiable from the diaries/cards/ glucometers

Patient's response

> Should be collected in diaries/cards/questionnaires

> Appropriate translation of the diaries/cards/questionnaires should be used

> Diaries/cards/questionnaires should be present in original at site

15.5 Adverse Events and Corrective Medications

> All Adverse events occurring during the course of study should be recorded with the respective start and stop dates

> Each adverse event should be recorded with the grade of severity

> Adverse events should be followed each time when the patient's visit takes place

> Patient should be evaluated for new adverse event(s) at every visit

> Medication once started by patient should be followed at every visit until it is stopped

> Dose/frequency should be documented

> Start and stop date should be clearly stated in the patient file

> Any change in the dosage/frequency should be documented

15.6 Drug Accountability

> Note down the number of units of each batch number of the drug(s) dispensed to the patient(s) at any visit

> Note down the number of units of each batch number of the drug(s) returned during each visit (if applicable)

> Any discrepancy (breakage/loss/damage should be properly documented

15.7 Progress Notes

> Patient's medical/progress notes should include details about the

    patient's medical condition and well-being across visits

➢ For unscheduled/telephonic visits, progress notes should be incorporated in the patient file

15.8 Patient's Status (ongoing)

➢ Patient's status/condition should be recorded on an ongoing basis

➢ If the patient is referred to another department/hospital; all the relevant details should be recorded in the source document

➢ If the patient is lost to follow-up, all communications/attempts to contact the patient should be mentioned in the patient file

All Source Documents should be archived for appropriate duration of time. If the institutional archival time is less than the trial requirements a special note should be mentioned on individual. Source Document and medical record section should be sensitized about it.

As trial patient requires a frequent follow-up, most of the investigators retain the source document of trial patients with them and a note in this regard is generally kept at the medical record section.

If electronic media is used for creating and/or storing source data proper care should be taken for ensuring the security, validation and back up control mechanism.

15.9 Tips on maintaining Source Document

☞ **Ensure that**

➢ The protocol number is mentioned on a patient file to highlight clinical trial participation

➢ The protocol number is present on the prescription form

➢ All entries in worksheets or patient files has date and initials of person making the entry

Proper access control should exist for the Source Document, which should be able to address "who did what" and "when it was done"

☞ **Document**

➢ The date patient gave consent, with the protocol number

➢ The consent process (whether the patient is literate or illiterate, who were the witness and which translation was used)

➢ The date the patient withdrew consent with reason (if any)

Voluntary consent is essential for protecting the rights, safety and well being of trial subject(s)

☞ **Make entries of**

➢ The number of units of each batch number of the investigational product dispensed to the patient(s) at scheduled visits

➢ The number of units of each batch number of the investigational product returned during each scheduled visit (if applicable)

➢ Any discrepancy (breakage/loss/damage)

Documentation of all the transaction of the study drug would lead to 100% drug accountability

☞ **Always make sure that**

➢ All the records of a patient are filed in one file or together

➢ If the patient is referred to another department/hospital, all the relevant records are included in the source document

➢ All investigational reports are duly signed and filed together in a chronological order

➢ All patient records/notes are together and in continuity

➢ Start and stop date for all adverse event(s) and corrective medication(s) are clearly stated in the patient file

Incomplete and inappropriate Source Document(s) can lead to significant audit issues

☞ **Find out**

➢ Where the source document(s) are kept once the study is over or after the patient's death

➢ How the source document(s) are kept (environmental protection from fire, flood, termite *etc.*)

All Source Documents are required to be archived for a specified period of time (10-15 years) after the completion of trial for the purpose of audit/inspection.

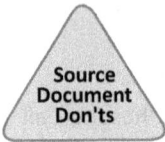

➢ Use of Xerox copy of CRF as Source Document

➢ Creation of trial specific Source Document

➢ Missing data/entries in the Source Document

➢ Changes to data questionable (no counter signatures of the person making the changes)

➢ Disorganized records with data for different entries of a patient kept in separate files

➢ Inappropriate filing of patient notes/report

➢ Messy documentation

➢ Lack of access control

➢ Source Document discarded after the trial is over

Summary Points

☑ Source Document should be able to tell the complete story and one should be able to reconstruct the entire trial simply on the basis of information captured in the Source Document.

☑ Use of CRFs as Source Document should be limited only to certain parameters like Quality of Life questionnaires, Evaluation scales, Patient demographics etc. and it should be mentioned in the Protocol.

☑ A good Source Document should be able to address: ICD process, pre-existing conditions and relevant medical history of the patient, laboratory reports and results, efficacy evaluations, adverse events and corrective medications, drug accountability, progress notes, ongoing status of the patient.

☑ Documentation of all the transaction of the study drug can lead to 100% drug accountability.

☑ Incomplete and inappropriate Source Document can lead to significant audit issues whereas a well maintained source document can help in the reconstruction of study at any given time point.

☑ All Source Documents are required to be archived for a specified period of time (10-15 years) after the completion of trial for the purpose of audit/inspection.

16

Management of Serious Adverse Event (SAE) and Regulatory Compliance

Serious Adverse Event (SAE) reporting constitutes one of the most important safety elements of any clinical trial. It is the responsibility of Investigator to report all the SAEs to the Sponsor/CRO and respective Ethics Committee. Sponsor in turn has the responsibility of reporting the same to the regulatory authority in a time bound manner and in compliance with applicable regulatory requirements.

An Adverse Event is any untoward medical occurrence in a clinical trial patient who has been administered a pharmaceutical product and which does not necessarily have a casual relationship with the treatment. An adverse event (AE) can therefore be any unfavorable and unintended sign (including an abnormal laboratory finding), symptom, or disease temporally associated with the use of a medicinal (investigational) product, whether or not related to the medicinal (investigational) product.

Serious Adverse Event (SAE) refers to any untoward medical occurrence that at any dose:

- ➤ results in death
- ➤ is life-threatening
- ➤ requires inpatient hospitalization or prolongation of existing hospitalization
- ➤ results in persistent or significant disability/incapacity
- ➤ is a congenital anomaly/birth defect

> ➤ is considered serious by the investigator for reasons other than those listed above

An SAE should meet the following four elements in order to qualify for a valid SAE:

1. an identifiable patient
2. an identifiable reporter
3. a suspect drug or biological product
4. an adverse event or fatal outcome

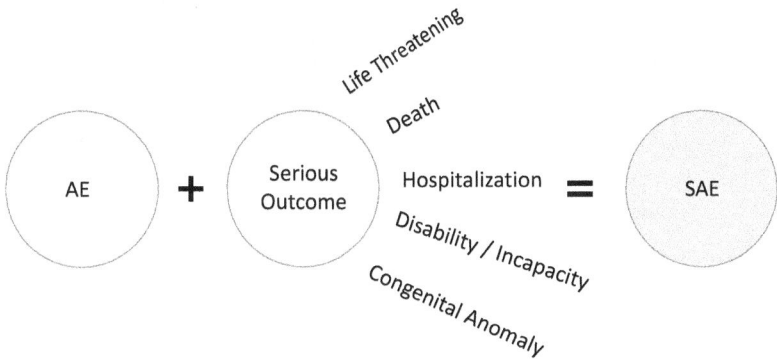

Figure 17. Criteria for a Valid SAE

In other words, if any of these basic elements remain unknown, a report on the incident should not be submitted to the regulatory authority because reports without such information make interpretation of their significance impossible in most instances.

The four basic elements are consistent with International Harmonization initiatives (International Conference on Harmonization; Guideline on Clinical Safety Data Management: Definitions and Standards for Expedited Reporting; ICH E2A document).

When a SAE Occur

> ➤ It is the responsibility of the investigational site to initiate a report

immediately upon becoming aware of it

➤ It is the responsibility of the Sponsor representative to submit an SAE report to Regulatory Agency with in the stipulated timeframe

16. 1 Investigator's Responsibilities on Safety Reporting

➤ All SAEs should be reported immediately to the sponsor except for those SAEs that the protocol or other document (*e.g.* Investigator's Brochure) identifies as not needing immediate reporting. The immediate reports should be followed promptly by detailed, written reports.

➤ The immediate and follow-up reports should identify subjects by unique numbers assigned to them rather than by the subject's names, personal identification numbers, and/or addresses

➤ The investigator should comply with the applicable regulatory requirement(s) related to the reporting of unexpected serious adverse drug reactions to the regulatory authority and the Ethics Committee

➤ Adverse events and/or laboratory abnormalities identified in the protocol as critical to safety evaluations should be reported to the sponsor according to the reporting requirements and within the time periods specified by the sponsor in the protocol

➤ For reported deaths, the investigator should supply the sponsor and the Ethics Committee with any additional requested information (*e.g.* autopsy reports and terminal medical reports)

16.2 Sponsor's Responsibilities on Safety Reporting

➤ Sponsor is responsible for the ongoing safety evaluation of the investigational product(s)

➤ The sponsor should promptly notify all concerned investigator(s) /institution(s) and the regulatory authority of findings that could affect adversely the safety of subjects, impact the conduct of the trial, or alter the Ethics Committee's approval to continue the trial

Reporting Timelines

➢ Investigator to Sponsor: Immediately (within **24 hours** of becoming aware of an SAE)

➢ Investigator to Ethics Committee: Within **24 hours** followed by a due-analysis report within 10 calendar days (Indian regulatory requirement)

SAE Impacts the safety of the patients hence quality data is essential. An attempt should be made to obtain complete and full information at the time of the initial/follow-up reporting. Complete case information includes information on:

➢ Patient Demographics
   - Gender, Age, Origin *etc.*

➢ Study Drug(s) Dosing Information
   - Date of first dose and
   - Date of last dose prior to SAE
   - Dosing units
   - Dosing schedule

➢ Study Drug(s) Indication(s) for Use

➢ Relevant Medical History
   - Relevant conditions that provide information or insight about events

➢ Relevant Clinical Information
   - Lab values and diagnostic test results that provide relevant information about the events or conditions

➢ Concomitant Medication
   - Medications received by the patient (other than study drugs) within 7 days of the SAE with stop/start dates and dosages

➢ Investigator Assessments and Rationale

- ➢ The sponsor should expedite the reporting to all concerned investigator(s)/ institution(s), to the Ethics Committee, and to the regulatory authority of all adverse drug reactions (ADRs) that are both serious and unexpected

- ➢ Such expedited reports should comply with the applicable regulatory requirement(s) and with the ICH Guideline for Clinical Safety Data Management: Definitions and Standards for Expedited Reporting

- ➢ The sponsor should submit to the regulatory authority all safety updates and periodic reports, as required by applicable regulatory requirements

It is the responsibility of sponsor(s) to train investigator(s)/site personnel on the accuracy and timeliness of serious adverse event reporting. Each serious adverse event should be followed-up until resolution and follow-up information should also be reported as soon as any additional information becomes available.

Though ICH-GCP requires regulatory reporting of death and life threatening events within 7 working days and other serious events within 15 working days of their occurance, Indian regulatory guidelines prescribes reporting of all serious adverse events within 10 calendar days.

In addition, Indian regulatory guidelines prescibes reporting to other participating sites within 14 calendar days. Further, Indian regulation also mandates the compensation in case of injury or death during clinical trial as per the requirements of Rule 122-DAB of Drugs and Cosmetics (First Amendment) Rules, 2013.

> Reporting Timelines

> Sponsor to Regulatory Authority

ICH-GCP Requirements:

- Death and Life threatening events: Within 7 working days

- All other events: Within 15 working days

Indian Regulatory Requirements:

- All events: Within 10 calendar days

> Sponsor to Other Participating Sites: Within 14 calendar days (Indian regulatory requirement)

It is the responsibility of Sponsor/CRO designee (Monitor) to verify the SAEs during the site monitoring visit from the source document. The prime objectives of SAE review is to ensure:

> Patient's protection

> Data accuracy and completeness

> Patient's continuation/discontinuation from the study

> Compliance with Ethics Committee reporting timelines

> Compliance with regulatory timelines and requirements

16.3 SAE Reporting Process Flow - Investigator's Responsibilities

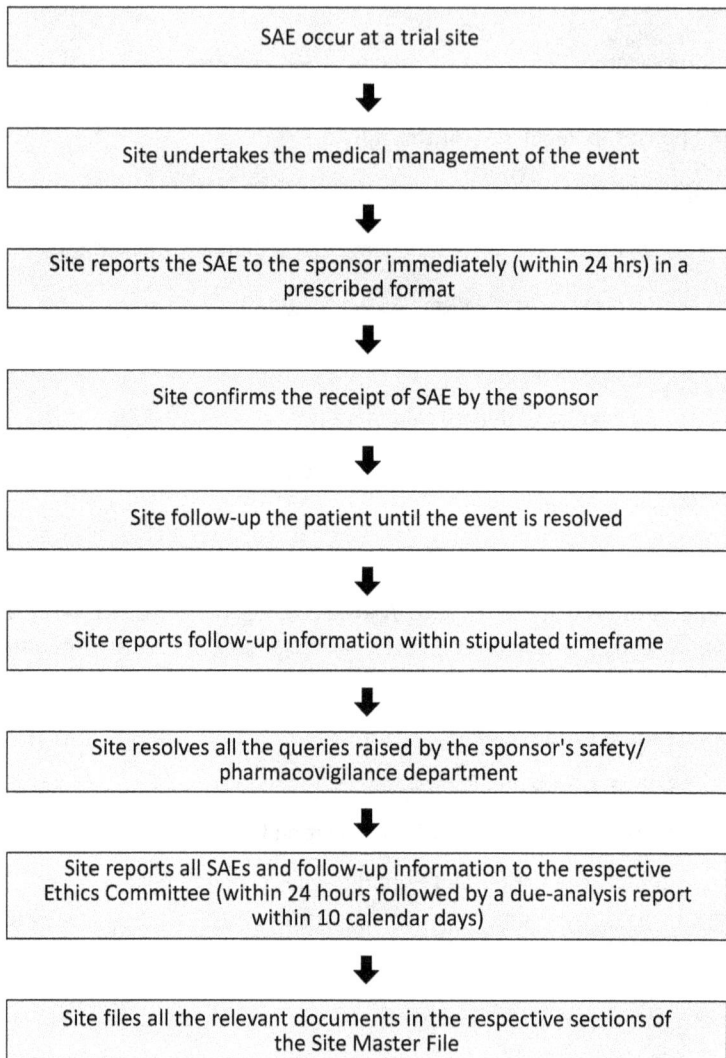

SAE occur at a trial site

⬇

Site undertakes the medical management of the event

⬇

Site reports the SAE to the sponsor immediately (within 24 hrs) in a prescribed format

⬇

Site confirms the receipt of SAE by the sponsor

⬇

Site follow-up the patient until the event is resolved

⬇

Site reports follow-up information within stipulated timeframe

⬇

Site resolves all the queries raised by the sponsor's safety/ pharmacovigilance department

⬇

Site reports all SAEs and follow-up information to the respective Ethics Committee (within 24 hours followed by a due-analysis report within 10 calendar days)

⬇

Site files all the relevant documents in the respective sections of the Site Master File

16.4 SAE Reporting Process Flow - Sponsor's Responsibilities

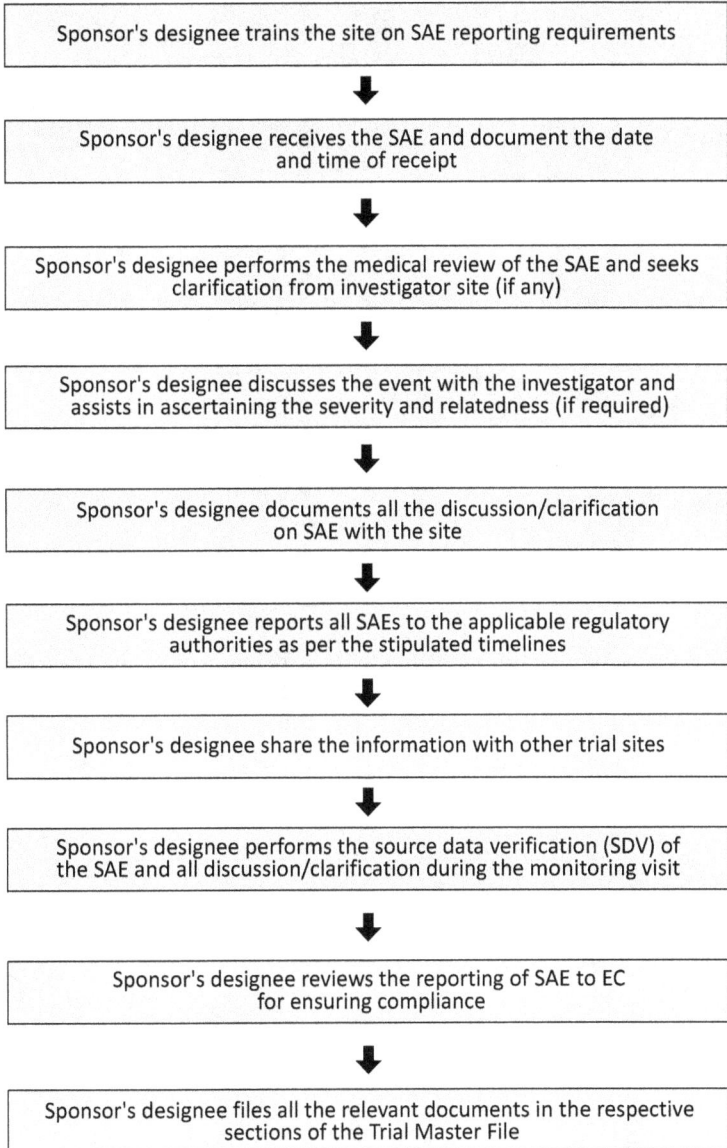

Sponsor's designee trains the site on SAE reporting requirements

⬇

Sponsor's designee receives the SAE and document the date and time of receipt

⬇

Sponsor's designee performs the medical review of the SAE and seeks clarification from investigator site (if any)

⬇

Sponsor's designee discusses the event with the investigator and assists in ascertaining the severity and relatedness (if required)

⬇

Sponsor's designee documents all the discussion/clarification on SAE with the site

⬇

Sponsor's designee reports all SAEs to the applicable regulatory authorities as per the stipulated timelines

⬇

Sponsor's designee share the information with other trial sites

⬇

Sponsor's designee performs the source data verification (SDV) of the SAE and all discussion/clarification during the monitoring visit

⬇

Sponsor's designee reviews the reporting of SAE to EC for ensuring compliance

⬇

Sponsor's designee files all the relevant documents in the respective sections of the Trial Master File

SAE REPORTING FORM (Appendix XI Format)

PROJECT NUMBER:

1. PATIENT DETAILS

Patient Number	Patient Initial	Gender	Age and/or Date of Birth	Weight (kg)	Height (cms)

2. SUSPECTED DRUG(S)

Generic Name	Indication (s)	Dosage Form and Strength	Dose Regimen (specify units)	Route of Administration	Starting Date	Stopping Date

3. OTHER TREATMENT(S)

4. DETAILS OF SUSPECTED ADVERSE DRUG REACTION(S)

5. OUTCOME
Information on recovery and any sequel; results of specific tests and/or treatment that may have been conducted. For a fatal outcome, cause of death and a comment on its possible relationship to the suspected reaction; Any post-mortem findings. Other information: anything relevant to facilitate assessment of the case, such as medical history including allergy, drug or alcohol abuse; family history; findings from special investigations *etc.*

6. DETAILS ABOUT THE INVESTIGATOR

Investigator Name	Address	Telephone Number(s)	Profession (Specify)

Date of Reporting the Event	Date of Reporting the Event to Ethics Committee Overseeing the Site

Signature of the Investigator	Date

Figure 18. SAE Reporting Form (Appendix XI Format of Schedule-Y)

Participating Investigators are informed of every possible related, unexpected case occurring at other trial site by a MedWatch/CIOMS Form/Appendix-XI format of Schedule-Y, detailing the case. MedWatch safety reports are sent to all investigators involved with the specific study or working with the specific compound, which is associated with a case meeting expedited criteria.

Upon receipt of a safety report (MedWatch/CIOMS/Appendix XI format of Schedule-Y), the investigators are required to notify their Ethics Committee about the same and document its review by signing the report.

Summary Points

- ☑ SAE reporting constitutes one of the most important safety elements of any clinical trial.

- ☑ SAE refers to any untoward medical occurrence that at any dose results in death, is life-threatening, requires inpatient hospitalization or prolongation of existing hospitalization, results in persistent or significant disability/incapacity, is a congenital anomaly/birth defect, is considered serious by the investigator for any other reasons.

- ☑ It is the responsibility of Investigator to report all the SAEs to the Sponsor within 24 hours of their occurrence.

- ☑ It is the responsibility of Investigator to report all the SAEs to the Ethics Committee within 24 hours followed by a due-analysis report within 10 calendar days.

- ☑ It is the responsibility of Sponsor to report all the SAEs to the Regulatory Authority within 10 calendar days of their occurrence.

- ☑ It is the responsibility of Sponsor to notify all concerned investigator(s)/institution(s) of the SAEs taking place in a clinical trial.

17

Investigational Product (IP) Accountability and Management

Investigational product refers to a pharmaceutical form of an active ingredient or placebo being tested or used as a reference in a clinical trial, including a product with a marketing authorization when used in a way different from the approved form, or when used for an unapproved indication, or when used to gain further information about an approved use.

It is the joint responsibility of the Sponsor and the Investigator(s) to maintain 100% accountability of the Investigational product at any given moment of time.

17.1 Investigator's Responsibilities:

- ➢ Handling and storage of Investigational Product
- ➢ Dispensing of Investigational Product to the patient(s)
- ➢ Documentation
- ➢ Accountability

17.2 Handling and Storage of Investigational Product

It is the responsibility of investigator(s) or designee to properly store the Investigational Product as per the instructions provided by the Sponsor/ CRO or as specified in the Protocol/ Investigator's Brochure/Drug Label.

This includes:

- ➢ Storing the IP at acceptable temperature conditions (*e.g.* room temperature, 2-8°C *etc.*)
- ➢ Storing the IP under appropriate storage conditions (*e.g.* protection from light, air, moisture *etc.*)
- ➢ Maintenance of temperature/humidity logs on a daily basis (recording of both minimum and maximum temperature)

17.3 Dispensing of Investigational Product to the Patient(s)

Investigator(s) or designee is responsible for dispensing the Investigational Product to the patients. While dispensing the Investigational Product to the patient(s), wherever applicable the investigator(s) or designee should comply with the reconstitution guidelines as specified in the Protocol/Investigator's Brochure/Label. Where the Investigational Product is to be given to the patients for consumption at home, clear instructions should be provided on the handling, storage, usage and accountability of the product.

17.4 Documentation

The following documents needs to be maintained by the investigator site:

- ➢ Document of shipment receipts
- ➢ Document of dispensing
- ➢ Documentation of temperature excursions (if any)
- ➢ Documentation of the return
- ➢ Documentation of destruction

17.5 Accountability

It is the responsibility of investigator(s) to maintain 100% accountability of both used and unused drug(s) for every trial. This is applicable for all the strengths and batches of Investigational Product. Appropriate documentation should be done for any breakage, loss, discrepancy *etc.* for the purpose of final accountability.

It is recommended that the accountability of Investigational Product at a site should not take more than 15 minutes. In order to have an ongoing accountability of all batches of Investigational Product it is important to design the accountability log in such a way that it captures all the transactions and shows the balance of used and unused medication at any time-point.

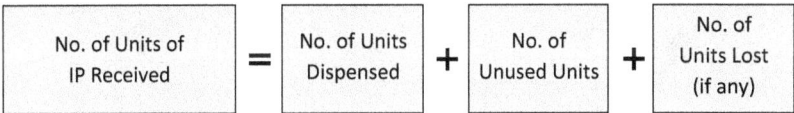

$$\text{No. of Units of IP Received} = \text{No. of Units Dispensed} + \text{No. of Unused Units} + \text{No. of Units Lost (if any)}$$

Figure 19. IP Accountability

Sponsor/CRO designee (Monitor) is responsible for designing the Master Drug Accountability Logs to capture all the required information that includes:

➢ Name and title of the trial

➢ Name and strength of Investigational Product

➢ Batch number

➢ Transactions (receipt, dispensing, returned, destroyed *etc.*)

➢ Patient number/visit number

➢ Balance of used and unused Investigational Product at a given time-point

➢ Signature of the personnel making the entries

➢ Comments

A separate Master Drug Accountability Log should be used for different types, strengths and batch number of Investigational Product(s).

If site undertakes the responsibility of destroying the used Investigational Product, destruction certificate should be maintained specifying the exact quantity and batch number of the material destroyed.

Protocol Code / Title:

Name of the Investigational Product:

Strength: **Batch Number:**

Sl. No.	Date	Transaction Type (R, D, RT¹, RT², O)	Patient No./ Visit No.	No. of Unused Units	No. of Used Units	Balance of Unused Units	Balance of Used Units	Comments	Signature

[**R** = Receipt, **D** = Dispensed, **RT¹** = Returned by the patient (if applicable), **RT²** = Returned to the Sponsor, **O** = Other]

Figure 20. Master Drug Accountability Log

17.6 Process Flow for IP Management at Investigator Site

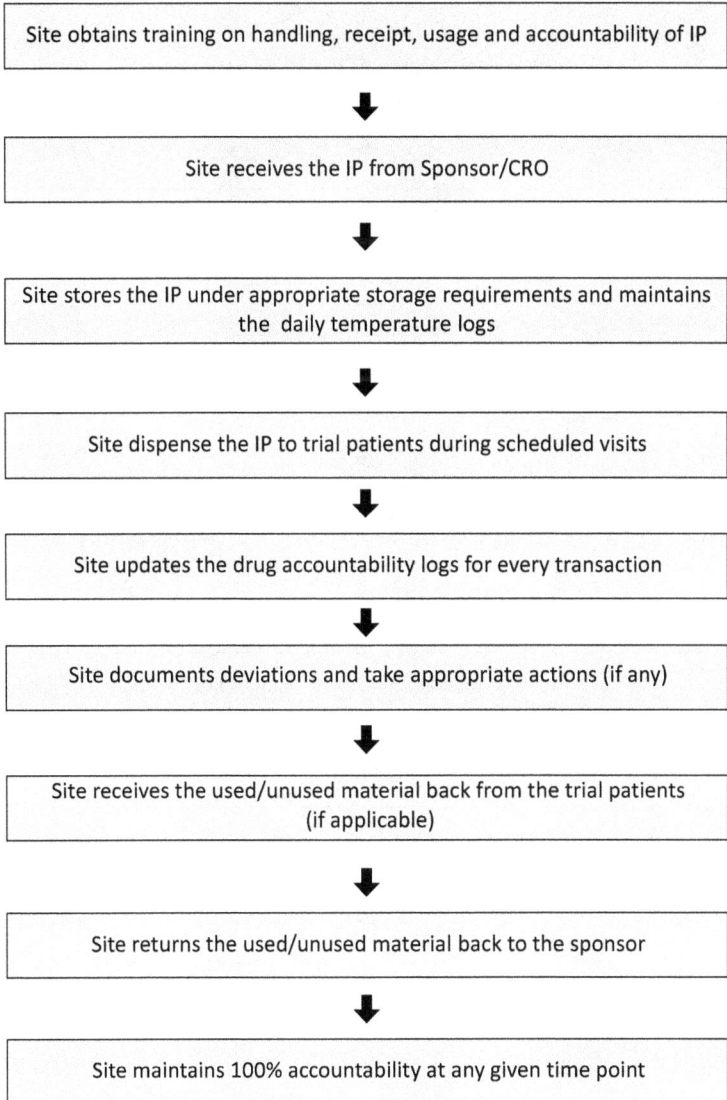

Site obtains training on handling, receipt, usage and accountability of IP

⬇

Site receives the IP from Sponsor/CRO

⬇

Site stores the IP under appropriate storage requirements and maintains the daily temperature logs

⬇

Site dispense the IP to trial patients during scheduled visits

⬇

Site updates the drug accountability logs for every transaction

⬇

Site documents deviations and take appropriate actions (if any)

⬇

Site receives the used/unused material back from the trial patients (if applicable)

⬇

Site returns the used/unused material back to the sponsor

⬇

Site maintains 100% accountability at any given time point

17.7 Process Flow for Investigational Product(s) Management by Trial Patients (wherever applicable)

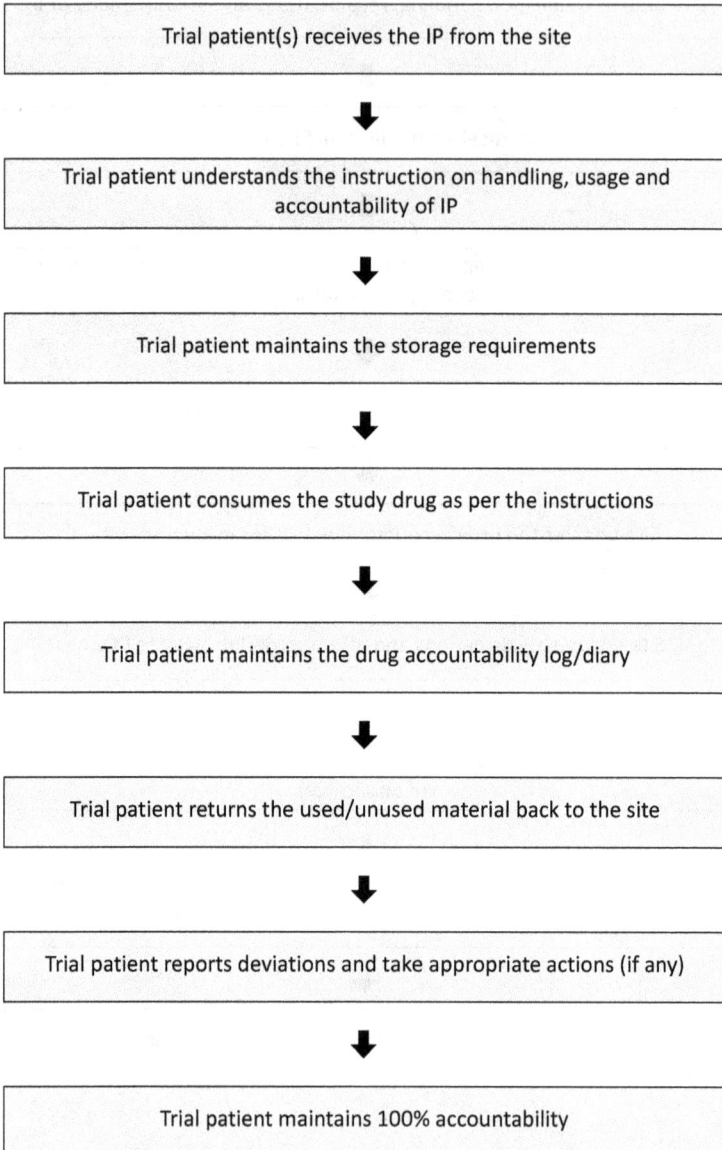

Trial patient(s) receives the IP from the site

↓

Trial patient understands the instruction on handling, usage and accountability of IP

↓

Trial patient maintains the storage requirements

↓

Trial patient consumes the study drug as per the instructions

↓

Trial patient maintains the drug accountability log/diary

↓

Trial patient returns the used/unused material back to the site

↓

Trial patient reports deviations and take appropriate actions (if any)

↓

Trial patient maintains 100% accountability

17.8 Tips on Investigational Product Accountability and Management

☞ **Ensure that**

➤ Regulatory Approval is available before initiating any clinical trial

➤ Test license is available for the import of IP

➤ A detailed training is provided to all the involved parties on handling, storage, reconstitution, dispensing and accountability of IP

Regulatory and GCP compliance is must in any clinical trial

☞ **Make entries of**

➤ The no. of units of each batch number of the IP dispensed to the patient(s) at each visit

➤ The no. of units of each batch number of the IP returned during each visit (if applicable)

➤ Any discrepancy (breakage/loss/damage)

Documentation of all the transactions of the IP would lead to 100% drug accountability

☞ **Always maintain the**

➤ Required temperature/humidity conditions for storage of IP

➤ Required storage conditions (protection from light/air *etc.*)

➤ Validated/calibrated temperature/humidity recording device (thermometer *etc.*)

Stability of IP is essential for protecting the rights/safety of trial subject(s) and integrity of trial data

☞ **Ensure that**

➤ IP is kept under proper access control

➤ Any deviation in storage condition is reported appropriately and the material is inspected for potency (if required)

➤ Temperature/humidity logs are maintained on a daily basis

Inappropriate handling of IP can lead to significant audit issue(s)

☞ **Make sure that at the end of the trial**

➤ Reconciliation of all used/unused IP is available at the site(s) level

➤ Reconciliation of all used/unused IP is available at the sponsor level

➤ Destruction certificate of IP is available

Lack of 100% reconciliation can jeopardize the trial data/outcome

---

Summary Points

☑ It is the joint responsibility of the Sponsor and the Investigator(s) to maintain 100% accountability of the Investigational product at any given time point.

☑ Documentation of all the transactions of the IP would lead to 100% drug accountability.

☑ It is the responsibility of Investigator/designee to maintain the temperature/humidity logs on a daily basis containing a recording of both minimum and maximum temperature.

☑ Master Drug Accountability Log should be designed in such a way that one log captures all the transactions and accountability.

☑ Inappropriate handling of IP can lead to significant audit issues and jeopardize the trial data/outcome.

18

Completion of Case Report Form (CRF) and Data Management

Once a trial is initiated at an investigator site and patients are recruited the next important step is to transcribe the data from the source document in to the Case Report Form (CRF). CRF refers to a pre-designed printed, optical, or electronic document used to record all the protocol-required information on each trial subject. Investigator can assign the duty of CRF completion to any of the study team member and generally this responsibility is assigned to the study coordinator.

Two different formats of CRF are available and include:

> ➤ Paper CRF (these are printed forms and site personnel have to make manual entries into it).

> ➤ Electronic CRF or e-CRF (these are electronic forms and site personnel have to transcribe the information directly into an electronic format using internet).

Though e-CRF is widely used now days, a Sponsor may choose to use the paper CRF for a specific trial.

Some of the key difference in Paper and e-CRF

Paper CRF	eCRF
Requires manual entry of data in pre-printed forms	Requires entry directly into an electronic format using internet
Occupies storage space of investigator site	No storage space required
Collection of paper CRF requires the Sponsor/ CRO designee to perform the monitoring visit	Data can be transcribed and uploaded as and when required
Data validation takes place after CRF collection and data queries (if any) are generated on a later date	Data validation takes place simultaneously and data queries (if any) can be resolved at the same time
Does not require the availability of a high-speed internet connection	Requires the availability of a high-speed internet connection
Data entry of the CRF is a rate limiting step in data cleaning	Data cleaning is faster

Table 3. Comparison Between Paper and e-CRF

It is the responsibility of investigator/designee to complete the CRF in an accurate and time-bound manner and this in turn is directly linked to the payment schedule of the study grant. Sponsor/CRO designee reviews the entries in the CRF *vis-à-vis* source document at every monitoring visit.

Steps of Data Management Process are as follows:

➢ Site fills the data from source document into the CRF

➢ CRFs are sent to the data management centre

➢ The logging (receipt, filing *etc.*) of CRF takes place at data management centre

➢ Data entry of CRF takes place on a computerized system containing the protocol specific validation plan. Usually double data entry is performed to avoid data entry errors

➢ Queries are generated based on Data Validation Plan

➢ Queries are sent to the sites

- ➤ Site personnel address the query and send the answered query back to data management centre. Usually the copy of answered query is filed along with the respective CRF page at the site

- ➤ Data management centre receives the answered query back from the site and resolves it in the data base

- ➤ Once the query is resolved the visit is declared as clean visit

- ➤ Data lock takes place when all the queries of all the patients are addressed and the entire patient visits are declared as clean

- ➤ Statistical analysis follows data lock

The data-outputs from statistical analysis are used in the clinical study report.

18.1 Process Flow for CRF Completion and Data Management at a Trial Site (Paper CRF)

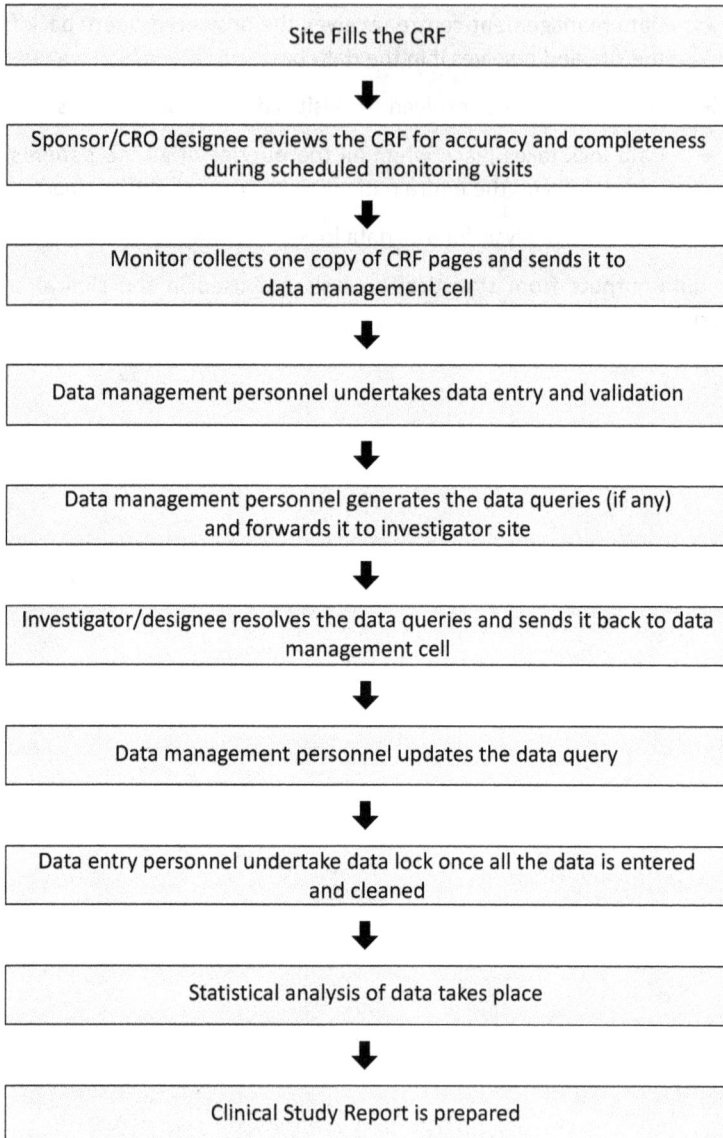

Site Fills the CRF

⬇

Sponsor/CRO designee reviews the CRF for accuracy and completeness during scheduled monitoring visits

⬇

Monitor collects one copy of CRF pages and sends it to data management cell

⬇

Data management personnel undertakes data entry and validation

⬇

Data management personnel generates the data queries (if any) and forwards it to investigator site

⬇

Investigator/designee resolves the data queries and sends it back to data management cell

⬇

Data management personnel updates the data query

⬇

Data entry personnel undertake data lock once all the data is entered and cleaned

⬇

Statistical analysis of data takes place

⬇

Clinical Study Report is prepared

18.2 Process Flow for CRF Completion and Data Management at a Trial Site (e-CRF)

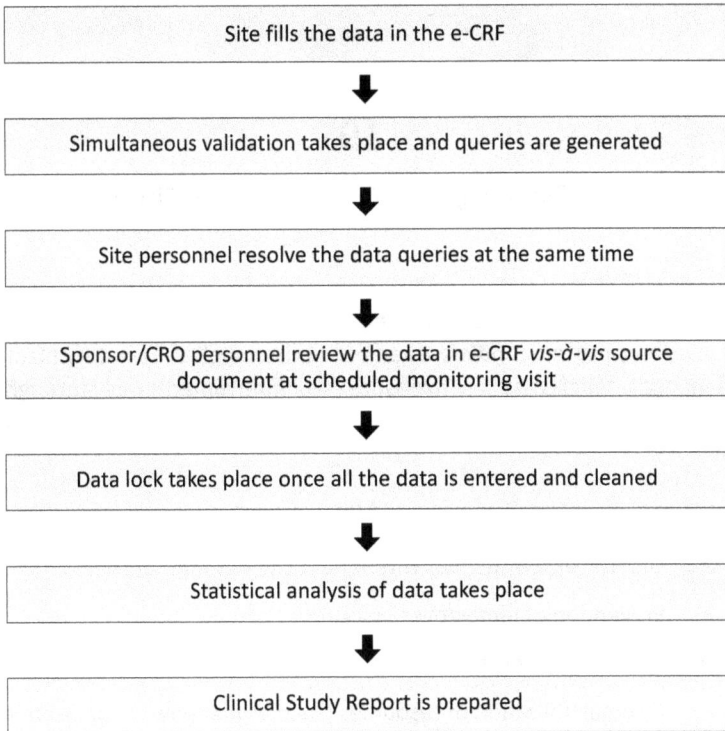

Site fills the data in the e-CRF

⬇

Simultaneous validation takes place and queries are generated

⬇

Site personnel resolve the data queries at the same time

⬇

Sponsor/CRO personnel review the data in e-CRF *vis-à-vis* source document at scheduled monitoring visit

⬇

Data lock takes place once all the data is entered and cleaned

⬇

Statistical analysis of data takes place

⬇

Clinical Study Report is prepared

Summary Points

☑ Two different formats of CRF are widely used, paper CRF and e-CRF.

☑ Collection of paper CRF requires the visit of Sponsor/CRO designee to the site.

☑ For e-CRF, data entry is made directly into an electronic format using internet and data validation takes place simultaneously.

☑ Data cleaning is faster in e-CRF compared to the paper CRF.

19

Inventory Planning and Management of Site Supplies

One of the responsibilities of a clinical study coordinator is to undertake the inventory planning and management of site supplies. Inventory planning and management is essential to ensure an uninterrupted supply throughout the duration of a clinical trial thereby leading to a smooth execution of a trial.

Objective of Inventory Planning and Management

- ➢ Uninterrupted supplies throughout the duration of trial
- ➢ Prevention of under/over stocking
- ➢ Cost-effectiveness
- ➢ Optimal utilization of resources (such as manpower, space *etc.*)

The various clinical trial materials that require Inventory planning, tracking and management include:

- ➢ Investigational Product(s)
- ➢ Lab Kits (if central lab is utilized)
- ➢ Thermometers
- ➢ Copies of Informed Consent Form and translations in vernacular language
- ➢ Case Report Forms
- ➢ Study specific device or equipments (if applicable)

➢ Packing Material *etc.*

Tips on Inventory Planning, Tracking and Management

➢ Read the protocol carefully to understand the critical junctures of the protocol such as dosage adjustment, study discontinuation *etc.*

➢ Keep sufficient supplies to meet the requirements of 6-8 weeks and order fresh supplies two weeks in advance

➢ Keep a track of patient enrolment and visits in order to calculate the requirement of investigation product and lab kits (if applicable) over a period of time

➢ Order the investigational product in small batches to avoid over-stocking

➢ Always add a buffer (~ 10%) for each study supply to take care of unforeseen circumstances

---

Summary Points

☑ Inventory planning and management is essential to ensure an uninterrupted supply throughout the duration of a clinical trial.

☑ A good inventory planning can avoid deviations that may arise due to insufficient supplies.

☑ A good inventory planning leads to an optimal utilization of space, manpower and resources.

20

Ongoing Correspondence with the Ethics Committee (EC)

After the initial approval of a clinical trial, it is the responsibility of investigator site to maintain the ongoing correspondence with the EC that has granted the initial approval.

The ongoing correspondence is required for submitting the:

- ➤ Reports of serious adverse event that has taken place at the site
- ➤ Safety reports (MedWatch/CIOMS Form/Appendix-XI format of Schedule-Y) for the suspected, unexpected serious adverse events that have taken place at other participating sites
- ➤ Amendment in the study protocol, informed consent form and other essential trial documents (if any)
- ➤ Updates of Investigator's Brochure
- ➤ Periodic study update report/ annual report as desired by the respective EC
- ➤ Protocol/process deviations
- ➤ Trial completion/suspension/termination report
- ➤ Clinical study report

While undertaking any correspondence with the EC, an investigator site should ensure that:

- ➤ Cover letter mentions the correct version number and date of the submitted documents

- ➤ Required number of copies are submitted to the EC as specified in the standard operating procedure of the EC

- ➤ Submission deadlines/timelines are met

- ➤ Acknowledgement of the receipt of document is obtained from the EC office

- ➤ Response letters from EC mentions the correct version number and date of the documents reviewed and/or approved

- ➤ Suggestions (if any) of EC is strictly followed

Summary Points

☑ All the SAEs and safety reports occurring in a clinical trial are required to be submitted to the EC within the stipulated timeframe.

☑ Any amendment in the essential study document is required to be approved by the EC before it becomes effective.

☑ Cover letter of all the correspondence to the EC should mention the correct version number and date of the documents submitted to EC.

21

Escalation, Management and Prevention of Violations/ Deviations

In order to ensure GCP and regulatory compliance it is important for an investigator site to document all the violations/deviations that have taken place during the conduct of a clinical trial. The violations/deviations can take place due to many reasons however, it is critical to document the violations/ deviations with a proper root cause analysis and rectification plan.

The importance of documenting violations/deviations is as follows:

- ➢ It provides an audit trail of what has happened, who did it and how it was resolved

- ➢ It can serve as very useful information at the time of regulatory inspections

- ➢ It can lead to process improvements if repeated violations/ deviations take place for a particular process

- ➢ Review of violations/deviations can be used as a training tool for new staff *etc.*

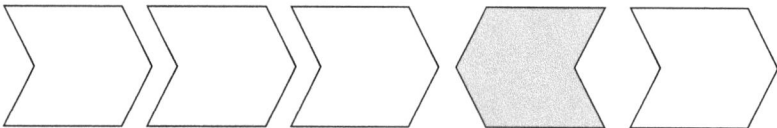

Figure 21. Violations/Deviations

21.1 Steps Involved in Escalation, Management and Prevention of Violations/Deviations

➢ Identification of violation/deviation with Root Cause and Rectification Analysis

➢ Documentation of violation/deviation with Action Plan

➢ Escalation of violation/deviation to the concerned authority

21.2 Identification of Violation/Deviation with Root Cause and Rectification Analysis

Any personnel involved in the conduct of a clinical trial can identify a violation/deviation however, this task is mostly done by Sponsor/CRO designee (Monitor). There are two broad categories of Violations/Deviations,

➢ Process Deviation: It refers to the deviation to the Standard Operating Procedures/Processes of the Sponsor, Institution or the regulatory guidelines

➢ Protocol Deviation: It refers to the deviation to the protocol schedule of events

Once a violation/deviation is identified the next step is to undertake a root cause and rectification analysis. The root cause and rectification analysis include:

➢ Description of the violation/deviation: what deviation has taken place?

➢ Root Cause of the violation/deviation: who is responsible for the deviation?

➢ Impact of the deviation on the conduct of study: does it affect the safety/efficacy data?

➢ Action plan: what action has taken place to rectify/prevent the violation/deviation?

➢ Responsibility: who is responsible for the action?

Only those violations/deviations are marked as significant that impacts the safety and efficacy data and are repeatable in nature.

21.3 Documentation of Violation/Deviation with Action Plan

Once the violation/deviation is identified the next step is to document it with proper action plan. The documentation of violation/deviation is generally done using a Deviation File Note. Investigator is required to sign and date all the deviations though it may have been caused by any other site team personnel.

21.4 Escalation of Violation/ Deviation to the Concerned Authority

After the documentation of violation/deviation the last step is to escalate it to the concerned authority (*e.g.* Sponsor/CRO, Ethics Committee, Regulatory Authority *etc.*).

Summary Points

☑ Documentation of violations/deviations provides an opportunity to generate an audit trail of what has happened, who did it and how it was resolved.

☑ Deviations/violations can serve as very useful information at the time of regulatory inspections.

☑ There are two broad categories of violations/deviations: process deviation and protocol deviation.

☑ Steps Involved in escalation, management and prevention of violations/deviations include : identification of the deviation with root cause and rectification analysis, documentation of the deviation with an action plan and escalation of the deviation to the concerned authority.

22

Clinical Trial Monitoring

Monitoring is the act of overseeing the progress of a clinical trial, and of ensuring that it is conducted, recorded, and reported in accordance with the protocol, Standard Operating Procedures (SOPs), Good Clinical Practice (GCP), and the applicable regulatory requirements.

The objective of the clinical trial monitoring is to ensure that:

> ➤ The rights and well being of human subjects are protected
> ➤ The reported trial data are accurate, complete, and verifiable from source documents
> ➤ The conduct of the trial is in compliance with the currently approved protocol, GCP and applicable regulatory requirement(s)

It is the responsibility of sponsor to ensure that the trials are adequately monitored. The sponsor should determine the appropriate extent and nature of monitoring. The determination of the extent and nature of monitoring should be based on considerations such as the objective, purpose, design, complexity, blinding, size, and endpoints of the trial.

In order to undertake the monitoring responsibility sponsor appoints a monitor for every trial who visits all the participating sites at a frequent interval and performs the onsite monitoring visit.

The critical elements of clinical trial monitoring include:

> ➤ Source Data Verification (SDV)
> ➤ Investigational Product (s) Accountability

- ➤ Informed Consent Form (ICF) Review

- ➤ Serious Adverse Events (SAEs) Review

- ➤ Review of Protocol Compliance

- ➤ Review of Regulatory Compliance

- ➤ Review of Investigator's Team Qualification and Training

- ➤ Review of Facility and Resources

- ➤ Review of Deviations and Actionable

- ➤ Review of Record Retention and Archival *etc*.

22.1 Source Data Verification (SDV)

SDV constitutes one of the prime elements of any monitoring visit and majority of time is generally spent on this activity. It includes verifying that:

- ➤ Source documents and other trial records are accurate, complete, kept up-to-date and maintained

- ➤ Data required by the protocol are accurately recorded in the source documents

- ➤ Any dose and/or therapy modifications and intercurrent illnesses are recorded appropriately

- ➤ Adverse events, concomitant medications and intercurrent illnesses are recorded with proper severity along with the start and stop dates

- ➤ Visits that the subjects fail to make, tests that are not conducted, and examinations that are not performed are clearly reported

- ➤ Laboratory reports, radiological investigations *etc*. are filed in original along with the progress notes

- ➤ All corrections, additions, or deletions are made, dated, explained (if necessary), and initialed by the investigator or by a member of the investigator's team who is authorized to make those changes

22.2 Investigational Product (s) Accountability

It includes verifying that:

- ➢ Storage conditions are acceptable, and sufficient inventory is available

- ➢ Investigational product(s) are supplied only to subjects who are eligible to receive it and at the protocol specified dose(s)

- ➢ Subjects are provided with necessary instruction on properly using, handling, storing, and returning the investigational product(s)

- ➢ All the transactions (receipt, use, return *etc.*) are controlled and documented adequately

- ➢ Disposition of unused investigational product(s) at the trial sites comply with applicable regulatory requirement(s) and are in accordance with the sponsor's requirements

- ➢ 100% accountability of all used/unused material is available at any given time point

22.3 Informed Consent Form (ICF) Review

It includes verifying that:

- ➢ Written informed consent is obtained before each subject's participation in the trial

- ➢ Appropriate translation (vernacular language) is provided to the subject for the ease of understanding

- ➢ An impartial witness/subject's legally acceptable representative was present while obtaining the informed consent from the illiterate patients

- ➢ A copy of the signed consent document is provided to each subject along with the emergency contact details

- ➢ Site copy is filed in the respective source file /case report form

22.4 Serious Adverse Events (SAEs) Review

It includes verifying that:

- ➤ All SAEs are appropriately reported within the stipulated time frame

- ➤ The investigator or the designee personally signs all SAEs

22.5 Review of Protocol Compliance

It includes verifying that:

- ➤ Investigator and the investigator's team are adequately informed about the protocol

- ➤ Investigator is enrolling the eligible patients only

- ➤ All trial patients follow the protocol schedule of events

- ➤ Any dose and/or therapy modifications are based on the protocol specifications

22.6 Review of Regulatory Compliance

It includes verifying that:

- ➤ Ethics Committee at a particular site operates as per the GCP, written standard operating procedures and the applicable regulatory requirement(s)

- ➤ Essential trial documents (Protocol, ICF and translations, Investigator Brochure, Patient diaries *etc.*) are approved by the respective EC

- ➤ Any amendment(s) to the essential documents is approved by the respective EC before becoming effective

- ➤ All SAEs are reported to the EC within the specified time frame

- ➤ Advertisement(s) used for enrolling the patients is approved by the EC

- ➤ Progress reports are submitted and the renewal of approval is taken within the specified time frame

> Suspension/cancellation/closure of the trial at the site is reported to the respective EC

22.7 Review of Investigator's Team Qualification and Training

It includes verifying that:

> Investigator's team qualification and training remains adequate through out the duration of trial

> Re-training is provided for the subsequent amendment(s) of the essential documents

> All new staff is trained on protocol and other elements before assigning specific responsibilities

> Investigator and the investigator's team are performing the specific trial functions, in accordance with the protocol and any other written agreement between the sponsor and the investigator/ institution, and have not delegated these functions to unauthorized individuals

> Roles and responsibilities (delegations) of individual team member is properly documented

22.8 Review of Facility and Resources

It includes verifying that the facilities including laboratories, equipments, drug storage, staff *etc.* are adequate to safely and properly conduct the trial and remains adequate throughout the duration of trial

22.9 Review of Deviations and Actionable

It includes verifying that:

> All the deviations (protocol, ICF, SAE, drug accountability, process *etc.*) are documented appropriately with root cause analysis

> Actionable taken to rectify the deviation(s) are adequate to prevent the recurrence of the detected deviations

> Learning is shared with all the team members and if deemed appropriate with the other investigator's sites involved in the trial

22.10 Review of Record Retention and Archival

It includes verifying that:

- ➤ All the trial records (master file, communication and logs, training binders *etc.*) are maintained up-to date with proper access control
- ➤ Records are readily retrievable as and when required
- ➤ All the trial records are archived as specified by the GCP and the applicable regulatory requirement(s)
- ➤ All the trial records are archived under proper environmental control (temperature, water, fire, pest *etc.*)

22.11 Process Flow for Clinical Trial Monitoring

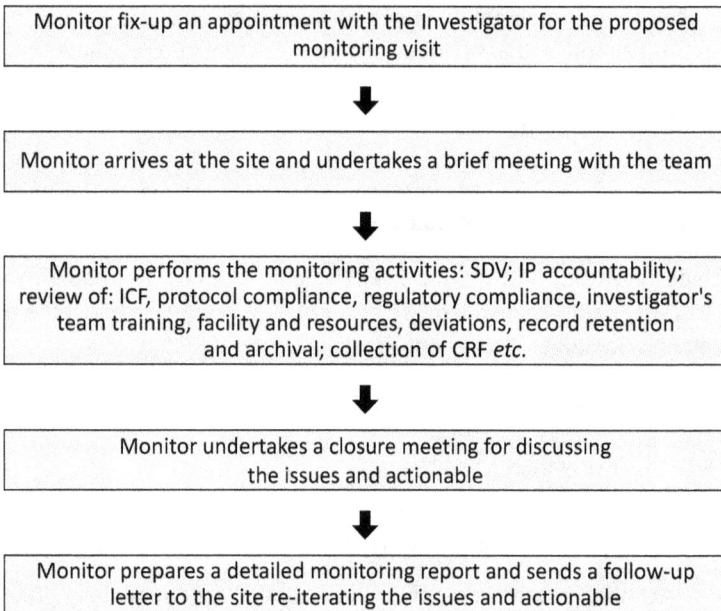

Monitor fix-up an appointment with the Investigator for the proposed monitoring visit

⬇

Monitor arrives at the site and undertakes a brief meeting with the team

⬇

Monitor performs the monitoring activities: SDV; IP accountability; review of: ICF, protocol compliance, regulatory compliance, investigator's team training, facility and resources, deviations, record retention and archival; collection of CRF *etc.*

⬇

Monitor undertakes a closure meeting for discussing the issues and actionable

⬇

Monitor prepares a detailed monitoring report and sends a follow-up letter to the site re-iterating the issues and actionable

Summary Points

☑ In order to undertake the monitoring responsibility sponsor appoints a monitor for every trial who visits all the participating sites at a frequent interval and performs the onsite monitoring visit.

☑ The critical elements of clinical trial monitoring includes: SDV, IP accountability, ICF review, SAE review, review of protocol and GCP compliance, review of investigator's team qualification and training, review of facility and resources, review of deviations review of record retention and archival.

☑ It is the responsibility of monitor to prepare a detailed monitoring report and forward the follow-up letter to the site re-iterating the issues and actionable.

23

Health Insurance Portability and Accountability Act (HIPAA) Privacy Rule

The Department of Health and Human Services (HHS) in US issued the Privacy Rule in December 2000 for safeguarding the privacy of individually identifiable health information.

Key Points:

> ➢ The Privacy Rule establishes minimum standards for protecting the privacy of individually identifiable health information. The Rule confers certain rights on individuals, including rights to access and amend their health information and to obtain a record of when and why their Personal Health Information (PHI) has been shared with others for certain purposes

> ➢ The Privacy Rule establishes conditions under which covered entities can provide researchers access to and use of PHI when necessary to conduct research. The Rule is not intended to impede research

> ➢ Compliance with the Privacy Rule is required on and after April 14, 2003, for most covered entities

The purpose of the Privacy Rule is to establish minimum standards for safeguarding the privacy of individually identifiable health information.

Covered entities, which must comply with the rule, are health plans, health care clearinghouses, and certain health care providers. Covered entities may not use or disclose PHI except as permitted or required under the provisions of the Privacy Rule.

The Privacy Rule recognizes that the research community has legitimate needs to use, access, and disclose individually identifiable health information to carry out a wide range of health research protocols and projects. In the course of conducting research, researchers may create, use, and/or disclose individually identifiable health information. The Privacy Rule protects the privacy of such information when held by a covered entity but also provides various ways in which researchers can access and use the information for research.

Protected Health Information - PHI is individually identifiable health information transmitted by electronic media, maintained in electronic media, or transmitted or maintained in any other form or medium.

Health Information - Any information, whether oral or recorded in any form or medium, that

> Is created or received by a health care provider, health plan, public health authority, employer, life insurer, school or university, or health care clearinghouse

> Relates to the past, present, or future physical or mental health or condition of an individual; the provision of health care to an individual; or the past, present, or future payment for the provision of health care to an individual

Individually Identifiable Health Information - Information that is a subset of health information, including demographic information collected from an individual, and

> Is created or received by a health care provider, health plan, employer, or health care clearinghouse

> Relates to the past, present, or future physical or mental health or condition of an individual; the provision of health care to an individual; or the past, present, or future payment for the provision of health care to an individual; and (a) that identifies the individual; or (b) with respect to which there is a reasonable basis to believe the information can be used to identify the individual

Summary Points

☑ The purpose of the HIPAA Privacy Rule is to establish minimum standards for safeguarding the privacy of individually identifiable health information.

☑ The Privacy Rule establishes conditions under which covered entities can provide researchers access to and use of PHI when necessary to conduct research.

☑ PHI is individually identifiable health information transmitted by electronic media, maintained in electronic media, or transmitted or maintained in any other form or medium.

24

Regulatory Inspections

Inspection refers to a systematic and independent examination of trial-related activities and documents to determine whether the evaluated trial-related activities were conducted, and the data were recorded, analyzed, and accurately reported according to the protocol, sponsor's Standard Operating Procedures (SOP), Good Clinical Practices (GCP) and the applicable regulatory requirements.

Since the Investigational New Drug Regulations went into effect in 1963, the Food and Drug Administration (FDA) has exercised oversight of the conduct of studies with regulated products. The Bioresearch Monitoring Program was established in 1977 by a task force that included representatives from the drug, biologic, devices, veterinary drug and food areas.

Compliance programs were developed to provide uniform guidance and specific instruction for inspections of clinical investigators, sponsors, contract research organizations, biopharmaceutical laboratories (in-vivo bio-equivalence), institutional review boards and non-clinical laboratories.

The purpose of the bioresearch-monitoring program is to assure the quality and integrity of data submitted to FDA to demonstrate the safety and efficacy of regulated products, and to determine that human rights and the welfare of human and animal research subjects are adequately protected. The compliance to regulations is assessed through audit procedures.

The various stakeholders that come under purview of Regulatory Inspections include:

> ➤ Sponsor(s)/CRO(s)

> Investigator(s)

> IRB/IEC/EC

24.1 Sponsor(s)/ CRO(s)

Regulations that govern the proper conduct of clinical studies establish specific responsibilities of sponsors for ensuring:

> the proper conduct of clinical studies

> the protection of the rights and welfare of subjects of clinical studies

Sponsors may transfer responsibility for any or all of the obligations to Contract Research Organizations (CROs). Under the regulations such transfer of responsibility are permitted by written agreement. Responsibilities that are not specified in a written agreement are not transferred. When operating under such agreements, the CROs are subject to the same regulatory actions as sponsors.

All inspections of sponsors, CROs, and monitors are conducted without prior notification unless otherwise instructed by the assigning Center.

Inspections are conducted to determine:

> How sponsors assure the validity of data submitted to them by clinical investigators

> The adherence of sponsors, CROs, and monitors to applicable regulations

Each inspection includes a detailed analysis of the practices and procedures of Sponsor/ CRO through:

> Organization and Personnel

> Selection and Monitoring of Clinical Investigators

> Selection of Monitors

> Monitoring Procedures and Activities

> Adverse Experience/Effects Reporting

> Data Collection and Handling

> Record Retention

> Automated Entry of Clinical Data (if applicable)
> Test Article (Investigational Agent)
> Sample Collection

Establishment Inspection Reports (EIR) classifications:

> **No Action Indicated (NAI)** - No objectionable conditions or practices were found during an inspection

> **Voluntary Action Indicated (VAI)** - Objectionable conditions or practices were found, but the agency is not prepared to take or recommend any administrative or regulatory action

> **Official Action Indicated (OAI)** - Regulatory and/or administrative actions will be recommended

24.2 Investigator Site (s)

Physicians and other qualified experts ("clinical investigators") are required to comply with applicable regulations intended to ensure the integrity of clinical data on which product approvals are based and to help protect the rights, safety, and welfare of human subjects.

Regulatory Inspection of Clinical Investigator(s) involves a comparison of the practices and commitments made in the applicable regulations. The nature of these inspections makes unannounced visits to the clinical investigator impractical. However, the time span between initial contact and actual inspection is kept as short as possible.

The inspection includes a comparison of the data submitted to the sponsor with supporting data (original records) at the site. Also the site personnel are interviewed to determine who did what and how it was done.

Documentation review is done to establish that research was conducted under proper authority, rights/safety/well-being of research subject were protected and data supports the conclusions.

FDA can disqualify a clinical investigator if he/she has repeatedly or deliberately failed to comply with applicable regulatory requirements or the clinical investigator has repeatedly or deliberately submitted false information to the sponsor. A disqualified clinical investigator is not eligible to receive investigational drugs, biologics, or devices.

Establishment Inspection Reports (EIR) classifications:

 ➢ **No Action Indicated (NAI)** - No objectionable conditions or practices were found during an inspection

 ➢ **Voluntary Action Indicated (VAI)** - Objectionable conditions or practices were found, but the agency is not prepared to take or recommend any administrative or regulatory action

 ➢ **Official Action Indicated (OAI)** - Regulatory and/or administrative actions will be recommended

24.3 Ethics Committee (EC)

FDA periodically inspects each EC that reviews research of FDA regulated products. These inspections are either surveillance or directed.

Surveillance Inspections

 ➢ Initial Inspection: The assigning Center provides evidence of FDA jurisdiction over the EC, the name and address of the institution, and when available, the name of a contact person at the EC

 ➢ Subsequent Inspections: Those IRBs found to be in full compliance (NAI) or with minor deficiencies (VAI) will usually be assigned for re-inspection in 5 years to determine their continued compliance with the regulations. Those ECs found to have major deficiencies will usually be assigned for re-inspection within one year to confirm that adequate corrections have been made

Directed Inspection

A "directed" inspection may be assigned when the assigning center receives information that calls into question the EC's practices. A directed inspection may be limited to one area of concern or assigned to cover the entire compliance program.

Establishment Inspection Reports (EIR) classifications:

 ➢ **No Action Indicated (NAI)** - No objectionable conditions or practices were found during an inspection.

➢ **Voluntary Action Indicated (VAI)** - Objectionable conditions or practices were found, but the agency is not prepared to take or recommend any administrative or regulatory action.

➢ **Official Action Indicated (OAI)** - Regulatory and/or administrative actions will be recommended.

24.4 Regulatory Inspection Process (US-FDA)

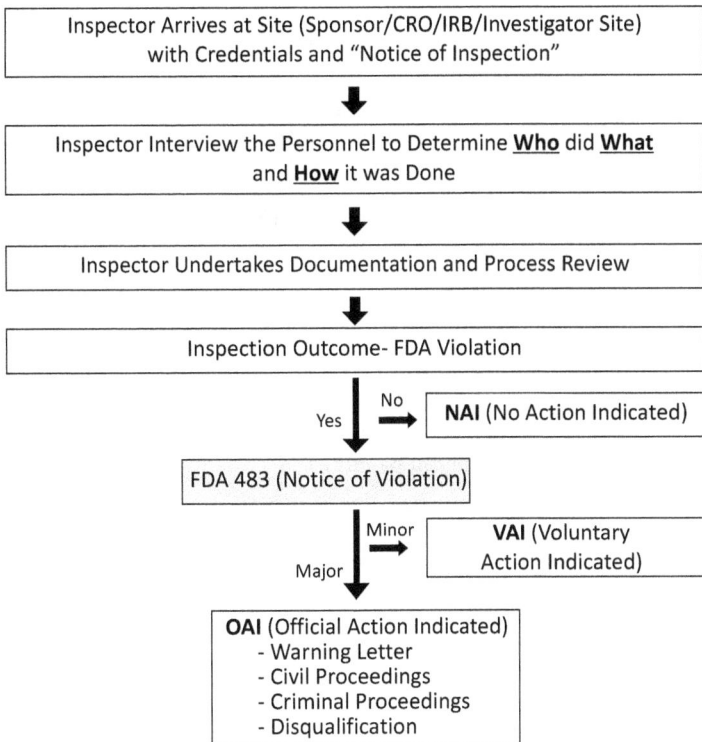

Figure 22. FDA Inspection Process

Summary Points

☑ Inspection refers to a systematic and independent examination of trial-related activities and documents to determine whether the evaluated trial-related activities were conducted, and the data were recorded, analyzed, and accurately reported according to the protocol, sponsor's standard operating procedures (SOP), Good Clinical Practices (GCP) and the applicable regulatory requirements.

☑ Regulatory inspection can take place for Sponsor, CRO, Investigator and EC.

☑ Inspection report is classified as NAI, VAI and OAI.

☑ All inspections of sponsors, CROs, and monitors are conducted without prior notification unless otherwise instructed by the assigning Center.

☑ FDA can disqualify a clinical investigator if he/she has repeatedly or deliberately failed to comply with applicable regulatory requirements. A disqualified clinical investigator is not eligible to receive investigational drugs, biologics, or devices.

☑ Inspections of ECs can be either surveillance or directed.

25

Site Close-out

Site close-out refers to closing trial sites after a clinical trial has been completed or suspended/ terminated. Site close-out activity is performed once a clinical trial is completed and the required data has been collected from the sites. However, in some cases a trial is suspended or terminated due to safety or efficacy concerns based on the results of interim analysis. In such cases, the site close-out visit is performed once the decision is taken to suspend/terminate the trial.

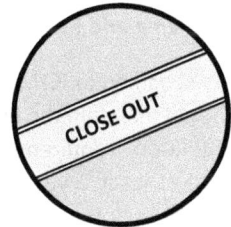

Close-out of Investigator Sites

It is the responsibility of Sponsor/CRO designee to notify the investigator site (s) of the site close-out visit date and pending tasks that needs to be completed before the close-out visit. Following activities are performed by the Sponsor/CRO designee at the site close-out visit:

> ➤ Return of any equipment leased or loaned by the Sponsor

> ➤ Review of all essential documents to be present at trial closure

> ➤ Review of pending data queries and its resolution

> ➤ Review of SAEs and follow-up reports for completion

> ➤ Review of master drug accountability logs for 100% reconciliation

> ➤ Review of final report to Ethics Committee

> Review of any outstanding payments and reconciliation of the study grants

The investigators are also reminded of

> Their archiving responsibilities as stated in Clinical Trial Agreement

> Regulatory audits and inspection

> Clinical study report process and publication policies *etc.*

A site close-out report is prepared for all participating sites and filed in their respective files.

Archiving and Retention of Essential Trial Documents

As specified in ICH-GCP, the sponsor as well as the investigator/institution should maintain the essential trial documents in accordance with applicable regulatory requirements. Essential study documents should be retained until at least 2 years after the last approval of a marketing application in an ICH region and until there are no pending or contemplated marketing applications in an ICH region or at least 2 years have elapsed since the formal discontinuation of clinical development of the investigational product. However, these documents should be retained even longer if required by applicable regulatory requirements or else agreed with the sponsor.

Summary Points

☑ Site close-out is done once a trial is completed, suspended or terminated.

☑ Sponsor/CRO designee reviews the availability all the essential documents required to be present at the time of site closure for ensuring regulatory compliance.

☑ Site close-out is documented by means of a written site close-out report.

26

Preparation of Clinical Study Report and Trial Publication(s)

26. 1 Clinical Study Report (CSR)

It is a written description of a trial on any therapeutic, prophylactic, or diagnostic agent conducted in human subjects, in which the clinical and statistical description, presentations, and analyses are fully integrated into a single report.

The structure and content of CSR as prescribed by ICH-GCP is as follows:

1. Title Page

2. Synopsis

3. Table of Contents for the Individual Clinical Study Report

4. List of Abbreviations and Definition of Terms

5. Ethics

    5.1   Independent Ethics Committee (IEC)

    5.2   Ethical Conduct of the Study

    5.3   Patient Information and Consent

6. Investigators and Study Administrative Structure

7. Introduction

8. Study Objectives

9.   Investigational Plan

   9.1   Overall Study Design and Plan-Description

   9.2   Discussion of Study Design

   9.3   Selection of Study Population

      9.3.1   Inclusion criteria

      9.3.2   Exclusion criteria

      9.3.3   Removal of patients from therapy or assessment

   9.4   Treatments

      9.4.1   Treatments administered

      9.4.2   Identity of investigational product(s)

      9.4.3   Method of assigning patients to treatment groups

      9.4.4   Selection of doses in the study

      9.4.5   Selection and timing of dose for each patient

      9.4.6   Blinding

      9.4.7   Prior and concomitant therapy

      9.4.8   Treatment compliance

   9.5   Efficacy and Safety Variables

      9.5.1   Efficacy and safety measurements

      9.5.2   Appropriateness of measurements

      9.5.3   Primary efficacy variable(s)

      9.5.4   Drug concentration measurements

   9.6   Data Quality Assurance

   9.7   Statistical Methods Planned in the Protocol and Determination of Sample Size

      9.7.1   Statistical and analytical plans

      9.7.2   Determination of sample size

12. Safety Evaluation

    12.1 Extent of Exposure

    12.2 Adverse Events (AEs)

        12.2.1   Brief summary of adverse events

        12.2.2   Display of adverse events

        12.2.3   Analysis of adverse events

        12.2.4   Listing of adverse events by patient

    12.3 Deaths, Other Serious Adverse Events, and Other Significant Adverse Events

        12.3.1   Listing of deaths, other serious adverse events, and other significant adverse events

            12.3.1.1   Deaths

            12.3.1.2   Other Serious Adverse Events

            12.3.1.3   Other Significant Adverse Events

        12.3.2   Narratives of deaths, other serious adverse events, and certain other significant adverse events

        12.3.3   Analysis and discussion of deaths, other serious adverse events, and other significant adverse events

    12.4 Clinical Laboratory Evaluation

        12.4.1   Listing of individual laboratory measurements by patient and each abnormal   laboratory value

        12.4.2   Evaluation of each laboratory parameter

            12.4.2.1   Laboratory Values Over Time

            12.4.2.2   Individual Patient Changes

            12.4.2.3   Individual Clinically Significant Abnormalities

    12.5 Vital Signs, Physical Findings, and Other Observations Related to Safety

    12.6 Safety Conclusions

13. Discussion and Overall Conclusions

14. Tables, Figures and Graphs Referred to But not Included in the Text

   14.1 Demographic Data

   14.2 Efficacy Data

   14.3 Safety Data

      14.3.1   Displays of adverse events

      14.3.2   Listings of deaths, other serious and significant adverse events

      14.3.3   Narratives of deaths, other serious and certain other significant adverse events

      14.3.4   Abnormal laboratory value listing (each patient)

15. Reference List

16. Appendices

   16.1 Study Information

      16.1.1   Protocol and protocol amendments

      16.1.2   Sample case report form (unique pages only)

      16.1.3   List of IECs or IRBs (plus the name of the committee Chair if required by the regulatory authority)

      16.1.4   List and description of investigators and other important participants in the study, including brief (1 page) CVs or equivalent summaries of training and experience relevant to the performance of the clinical study

      16.1.5   Signatures of principal or coordinating investigator(s) or sponsor's responsible medical officer, depending on the regulatory authority's requirement.

      16.1.6   Listing of patients receiving test drug(s)/investigational product(s) from specific batches, where more than one batch was used

      16.1.7   Randomization scheme and codes (patient identification and treatment assigned)

      16.1.8   Audit certificates (if available)

26.2 Publication

In this era of evidence-based medicine, one always strives to review the published literature in order to make opinion about a particular drug or a therapy. However many clinical trials never get published, which means that published literature may give a very inadequate picture of what is known about a drug.

Publication is the final stage of research and it is unethical to not publish the research work. Publication means presenting the research so that it is made publicly available, and includes enough detail so that its reliability and validity can be fairly assessed.

All the scientific papers and publications follow a standard format which is as follows :

- ➤ Title Page
- ➤ Abstract
- ➤ Introduction
- ➤ Patients and Methods
- ➤ Results
- ➤ Discussion
- ➤ References
- ➤ Tables

Title page:

Title page of the article should contain the following information

- ➤ The title of the article.
- ➤ Authors' names and institutional affiliations
- ➤ The name of the department(s) and institution(s) to which the work should be attributed
- ➤ Disclaimers, if any
- ➤ Corresponding authors
- ➤ Source(s) of support in the form of grants, equipment, drugs, or all of these
- ➤ Word counts
- ➤ The number of figures and tables

Abstract

An abstract should follow the title page. The abstract should provide the context or background for the study and should state the study's purposes, basic procedures, main findings, and conclusions. It should emphasize new and important aspects of the study or observations.

- ➢ Be concise and report only essential data
- ➢ Follow guidelines of meeting or journal

Introduction:

This section provides a context or background for the study (*i.e.*, the nature of the problem and its significance).

Patient and Methods:

This section should provide details on:

- ➢ Eligibility criteria (inclusion, exclusion)
- ➢ Treatment regimen(s) and key dose modification guidelines
- ➢ Key study procedures (including criteria for efficacy endpoints and toxicity grading), tests, investigations
- ➢ Statistics; study design, hypothesis, methods

Results:

This section should provide sufficient details on the findings of the study. Results should be presented using the tables and figures for the ease of interpretation.

Discussion:

This section should provide details on:

- ➢ Key outcomes of your study *vis-à-vis* existing literature.

References:

This section should list all the references used in preparing the publication in a standard format.

Tables and Figures

These should be appended along with the publication.

26.3 Useful Publication Tips:

- ➢ Decide your target Journal beforehand and reads the 'Instructions for Authors' carefully before drafting a publication
- ➢ Refer to the instructions for drafting each section of the publication
- ➢ Insert a comma wherever there is a slight pause between words or phrases in the spoken sentence
- ➢ Insert a semicolon between two parts of a sentence
- ➢ Use a colon to introduce an explanation or an example of something
- ➢ Use italics for emphasis and bold for strong emphasis
- ➢ Don't start sentences with because, since, or as
- ➢ Use while and since to refer to time
- ➢ Make sure you write well-formed sentences, and keep their structure simple
- ➢ Organize the content to give the feeling of a good story while reading
- ➢ Arrange the references as per the style recommended in the instructions
- ➢ Address the queries of reviewers (if any) within the stipulated time-frame

Summary Points

☑ CSR is a written description of a trial on any therapeutic, prophylactic, or diagnostic agent conducted in human subjects, in which the clinical and statistical description, presentations, and analyses are fully integrated into a single report.

☑ Publication refers to presenting the research so that it is made publicly available, and includes enough detail so that its reliability and validity can be fairly assessed.

Appendix-1. Tips on Essential Trial Documents

1 Protocol

➢ Protocol must contain all the ICH-GCP required elements

➢ A version date and a version number should identify the approved protocol

➢ Regulatory and EC approval must be obtained for each clinical trial protocol

➢ Version control should be maintained for all subsequent amendments

➢ A tracking log should be maintained to record version(s) control

2 Informed Consent Form (ICF)

➢ ICF must contain all the ICH-GCP required elements

➢ A version date and a version number should identify each ICF

➢ Translation of ICF in vernacular languages must be approved by Ethics Committee (EC)

➢ Only the EC approved version of ICF should be administered to the patients

➢ Version control should be maintained for all subsequent amendments

➢ A tracking log should be maintained to record version(s) control

➢ ICF should be obtained before non-routine screening procedures are performed and/or before any change in the subject's current medical therapy is made for the purpose of the clinical trial

➢ Investigator or designee should personally obtain the ICF from the subject

➢ Subject should receive a copy of the signed ICF

3 Investigator's Brochure (IB)

- ➢ IB must contain all the ICH-GCP required elements
- ➢ A version date and a version number should identify each IB
- ➢ ERB must review each version of IB
- ➢ IB should be updated on a regular interval to include all new data on the Investigational product
- ➢ Previous version of IB should be destroyed once the updated version is available

4 Case Report Form (CRF)

- ➢ CRF should be designed to include all the required data
- ➢ CRF should preferably be made of NCR (no carbon required) paper

5 Source Document (SD)

- ➢ All entries in worksheets or patient files should have the date and initials of person making the entry
- ➢ All the records of a patient should be filed in one file or together. If the patient is referred to another department/hospital, all the relevant records should be included in the source document
- ➢ Start and stop date for all adverse event(s) and corrective medication(s) should be clearly stated in the patient's source document
- ➢ Environmental control (protection from fire, flood, termite *etc.*) must be maintained throughout the duration of archival

6 Regulatory Approval

- ➢ Regulatory approval must be obtained prior to initiating any clinical trial in India
- ➢ Regulatory approval must contain the duration of approval
- ➢ Regulatory approval must be obtained for all subsequent amendment(s)

7 EC Approval

- ➤ EC approval should include the name and version(s) of the documents reviewed for granting approval
- ➤ EC approval must contain signature, date and seal of chairperson; list of voting members; and list of members who were absent
- ➤ EC approval must contain the duration of approval
- ➤ EC approval must be obtained prior to initiating a clinical trial at any site
- ➤ EC approval must be obtained for all subsequent amendment(s)

8 Advertisement

- ➤ All trial related advertisement must be approved by EC
- ➤ Wordings of advertisement should be such that it does not coerce the patient(s) to participate in a clinical trial

9 Financial Agreements

- ➤ All trial related financial agreement should be in compliance with the individual institution and the local laws
- ➤ The hospital administration and the EC should be made aware of the financial aspect of the trial
- ➤ All trial related grants/payments should be made in accordance with the financial agreement

10 Insurance Statement

- ➤ Sponsor should provide the insurance statement prior to initiating the trial at a particular site
- ➤ Insurance statement should include the compensation clause for all trial related injuries

11 Curriculum Vitae (CV)

- ➤ CV should contain the most updated information
- ➤ CV must be obtained from all the concerned personnel prior to initiating a clinical trial
- ➤ CV should be personally signed and dated by the concerned personnel

12 Laboratory Reference Range

- ➤ Laboratory reference range must be obtained prior to initiating the clinical trial at a particular site
- ➤ It should be personally signed and dated by the concerned personnel

13 Monitoring Report

- ➤ Monitoring report should include all finding and issues with actionable and timelines
- ➤ Monitoring report should document all violations and protocol non-compliance

14 Investigational Product Accountability

- ➤ Investigational product(s) should be stored at required temperature/ humidity conditions
- ➤ Temperature/humidity logs should be maintained on a daily basis
- ➤ Investigational product should be kept under proper access control
- ➤ Any deviation in storage condition should be reported appropriately and the material should be inspected for potency (if required)
- ➤ Reconciliation of all used/unused Investigational Product(s) should be available at the site(s) level

➤ Reconciliation of all used/unused Investigational Product(s) should be available at the sponsor level

➤ Any loss/damage/breakage *etc*. should be properly documented

➤ Destruction certificate of Investigational Product(s) should be available at all levels

15 Certificate(s) of Analysis (COA)

➤ COA should be present for each batch and class of investigational product(s)

➤ COA should be available prior to initiating the clinical trial

16 Serious Adverse Event (SAE) Reporting

➤ An SAE should be reported only if it meets the requirements of a valid case (*i.e.* an identifiable patient; an identifiable reporter; a suspect drug or biological product; and an adverse event or fatal outcome)

➤ All SAEs must meet the reporting timelines as specified by the sponsor

➤ All the SAEs and follow-up reports at a particular site should be reported to respective EC

➤ All the valid SAE cases should be reported to applicable regulatory authority(ies) within the stipulated timeframe

17 Correspondence

➤ All correspondence should contain a date and an identifiable reporter

➤ All correspondence should be filed to provide an audit trail

18 Data Queries

➤ The designated personnel should sign all queries

➤ Individual query should be filed with the respective CRF page for which the query is generated

19 Clinical Study Report (CSR)

➤ CSR should be prepared irrespective of the trial outcome (positive or negative)

➤ CSR should be submitted to applicable regulatory bodies

Appendix-2. Structure and Content of Clinical Trial Protocol (ICH-GCP Required Elements)

1.1 General Information

1.1.1   Protocol title, protocol identifying number, and date. Any amendment(s) should also bear the amendment number(s) and date(s).

1.1.2   Name and address of the sponsor and monitor (if other than the sponsor).

1.1.3   Name and title of the person(s) authorized to sign the protocol and the protocol amendment(s) for the sponsor.

1.1.4   Name, title, address, and telephone number(s) of the sponsor's medical expert (or dentist when appropriate) for the trial.

1.1.5   Name and title of the investigator(s) who is (are) responsible for conducting the trial, and the address and telephone number(s) of the trial site(s).

1.1.6   Name, title, address, and telephone number(s) of the qualified physician (or dentist, if applicable), who is responsible for all trial-site related medical (or dental) decisions (if other than investigator).

1.1.7   Name(s) and address(es) of the clinical laboratory(ies) and other medical and/or technical department(s) and/or institutions involved in the trial.

1.2 Background Information

1.2.1   Name and description of the investigational product(s).

1.2.2   A summary of findings from nonclinical studies that potentially have clinical significance and from clinical trials that are relevant to the trial.

1.2.3 Summary of the known and potential risks and benefits, if any, to human subjects.

1.2.4 Description of and justification for the route of administration, dosage, dosage regimen, and treatment period(s).

1.2.5 A statement that the trial will be conducted in compliance with the protocol, GCP and the applicable regulatory requirement(s).

1.2.6 Description of the population to be studied.

1.2.7 References to literature and data that are relevant to the trial, and that provide background for the trial.

1.3 Trial Objectives and Purpose

A detailed description of the objectives and the purpose of the trial.

1.4 Trial Design

The scientific integrity of the trial and the credibility of the data from the trial depend substantially on the trial design. A description of the trial design, should include:

1.4.1 A specific statement of the primary endpoints and the secondary endpoints, if any, to be measured during the trial.

1.4.2 A description of the type/design of trial to be conducted (e.g. double-blind, placebo-controlled, parallel design) and a schematic diagram of trial design, procedures and stages.

1.4.3 A description of the measures taken to minimize/avoid bias, including:

(a) Randomization.

(b) Blinding.

1.4.4 A description of the trial treatment(s) and the dosage and dosage regimen of the investigational product(s). Also include a description of the dosage form, packaging, and labelling of the investigational product(s).

1.4.5   The expected duration of subject participation, and a description of the sequence and duration of all trial periods, including follow-up, if any.

1.4.6   A description of the "stopping rules" or "discontinuation criteria" for individual subjects, parts of trial and entire trial.

1.4.7   Accountability procedures for the investigational product(s), including the placebo(s) and comparator(s), if any.

1.4.8   Maintenance of trial treatment randomization codes and procedures for breaking codes.

1.4.9   The identification of any data to be recorded directly on the CRFs (i.e. no prior written or electronic record of data), and to be considered to be source data.

1.5 Selection and Withdrawal of Subjects

1.5.1   Subject inclusion criteria.

1.5.2   Subject exclusion criteria.

1.5.3   Subject withdrawal criteria (i.e. terminating investigational product treatment/trial treatment) and procedures specifying:
   (a)   When and how to withdraw subjects from the trial/ investigational product treatment.
   (b)   The type and timing of the data to be collected for withdrawn subjects.
   (c)   Whether and how subjects are to be replaced.
   (d)   The follow-up for subjects withdrawn from investigational product treatment/trial treatment.

1.6 Treatment of Subjects

1.6.1   The treatment(s) to be administered, including the name(s) of all the product(s), the dose(s), the dosing schedule(s), the route/ mode(s) of administration, and the treatment period(s), including the follow-up period(s) for subjects for each investigational product treatment/trial treatment group/arm of the trial.

1.6.2 Medication(s)/treatment(s) permitted (including rescue medication) and not permitted before and/or during the trial.

1.6.3 Procedures for monitoring subject compliance.

1.7 Assessment of Efficacy

1.7.1 Specification of the efficacy parameters.

1.7.2 Methods and timing for assessing, recording, and analysing of efficacy parameters.

1.8 Assessment of Safety

1.8.1 Specification of safety parameters.

1.8.2 The methods and timing for assessing, recording, and analysing safety parameters.

1.8.3 Procedures for eliciting reports of and for recording and reporting adverse event and intercurrent illnesses.

1.8.4 The type and duration of the follow-up of subjects after adverse events.

1.9 Statistics

1.9.1 A description of the statistical methods to be employed, including timing of any planned interim analysis(ses).

1.9.2 The number of subjects planned to be enrolled. In multicentre trials, the numbers of enrolled subjects projected for each trial site should be specified. Reason for choice of sample size, including reflections on (or calculations of) the power of the trial and clinical justification.

1.9.3 The level of significance to be used.

1.9.4 Criteria for the termination of the trial.

1.9.5 Procedure for accounting for missing, unused, and spurious data.

1.9.6 Procedures for reporting any deviation(s) from the original statistical plan (any deviation(s) from the original statistical plan should be described and justified in protocol and/or in the final report, as appropriate).

1.9.7 The selection of subjects to be included in the analyses (e.g. all randomized subjects, all dosed subjects, all eligible subjects, evaluable subjects).

1.10 Direct Access to Soure Data/Documents

The sponsor should ensure that it is specified in the protocol or other written agreement that the investigator(s)/institution(s) will permit trial-related monitoring, audits, IRB/IEC review, and regulatory inspection(s), providing direct access to source data/documents.

1.11 Quality Control and Quality Assurance

1.12 Ethics

Description of ethical considerations relating to the trial.

1.13 Data Handling and Record Keeping

1.14 Financing and Insurance

Financing and insurance if not addressed in a separate agreement.

1.15 Publication Policy

Publication policy, if not addressed in a separate agreement.

1.16 Supplements

(NOTE: Since the protocol and the clinical trial/study report are closely related, further relevant information can be found in the ICH Guideline for Structure and Content of Clinical Study Reports.)

Appendix-3. Informed Consent Document Review Checklist for ICH-GCP Required Elements

Sl. No.	Section/ Subsection	Statement	Present	Absent	NA
1.	ICH 4.8.10 (a)	That the trial involves research.			
2.	ICH 4.8.10 (b)	The purpose of the trial.			
3.	ICH 4.8.10 (c)	The trial treatment(s) and the probability for random assignment to each treatment.			
4.	ICH 4.8.10 (d)	The trial procedures to be followed, including all invasive procedures.			
5.	ICH 4.8.10 (e)	The subject's responsibilities.			
6.	ICH 4.8.10 (f)	Those aspects of the trial that are experimental.			
7.	ICH 4.8.10 (g)	The reasonably foreseeable risks or inconveniences to the subject and, when applicable, to an embryo, fetus, or nursing infant.			
8.	ICH 4.8.10 (h)	The reasonably expected benefits. When there is no intended clinical benefit to the subject, the subject should be made aware of this.			
9.	ICH 4.8.10 (i)	The alternative procedure(s) or course(s) of treatment that may be available to the subject, and their important potential benefits and risks.			

Sl. No.	Section/ Subsection	Statement	Present	Absent	NA
10.	ICH 4.8.10 (j)	The compensation and/or treatment available to the subject in the event of trial-related injury.			
11.	ICH 4.8.10 (k)	The anticipated prorated payment, if any, to the subject for participating in the trial.			
12.	ICH 4.8.10 (l)	The anticipated expenses, if any, to the subject for participating in the trial.			
13.	ICH 4.8.10 (m)	That the subject's participation in the trial is voluntary and that the subject may refuse to participate or withdraw from the trial, at any time, without penalty or loss of benefits to which the subject is otherwise entitled.			
14.	ICH 4.8.10 (n)	That the monitor(s), the auditor(s), the IRB/IEC, and the regulatory authority(ies) will be granted direct access to the subject's original medical records for verification of clinical trial procedures and/or data, without violating the confidentiality of the subject, to the extent permitted by the applicable laws and regulations and that, by signing a written informed consent form, the subject or the subject's legally acceptable representative is authorizing such access.			
15.	ICH 4.8.10 (o)	That records identifying the subject will be kept confidential and, to the extent permitted by the applicable laws and/ or regulations, will not be made publicly available. If the results of the trial are published, the subject's identity will remain confidential.			

Sl. No.	Section/ Subsection	Statement	Present	Absent	NA
16.	ICH 4.8.10 (p)	That the subject or the subject's legally acceptable representative will be informed in a timely manner if information becomes available that may be relevant to the subject's willingness to continue participation in the trial.			
17.	ICH 4.8.10 (q)	The person(s) to contact for further information regarding the trial and the rights of trial subjects, and whom to contact in the event of trial-related injury.			
18.	ICH 4.8.10 (r)	The foreseeable circumstances and/or reasons under which the subject's participation in the trial may be terminated.			
19.	ICH 4.8.10 (s)	The expected duration of the subject's participation in the trial.			
20.	ICH 4.8.10 (t)	The approximate number of subjects involved in the trial.			

Appendix-4. Clinical Trials in India: Dilemmas for Developing Countries

Published in The Monitor 2007; 21(2): 69-71

Clinical Research is an indispensable part of drug discovery process to ensure the safety and efficacy of any new drug. In today's global scientific era, clinical trials are the mainstay for bringing out newer and better drugs to the market. Although a set of robust guidelines are available that governs the conduct of clinical trials in any country, the conduct of clinical research is also looked upon as an area of humanitarian concern.

Various articles published recently in the professional and popular press enumerate the opportunities and challenges of conducting global clinical trials in India. However, the majority have been from the perspective of authors who have never conducted clinical trials in India themselves thereby presenting a biased view on this topic. Having worked as Principal Investigator for various global clinical trials in Medical Oncology, I would like to focus on some of the real time opportunities that have been largely negated due to a biased vision on clinical trials.

Country Background

A nation with more than 1 billion people, India has the second largest population in the world. Having gained its independence from British rule in 1947, its prime minister is the head of government and the president is the head of state. Internationally, India became a member of World Trade Organization (WTO) in 1995 and agreed to adhere to the product patent regime by 2005. As a result, the global pharmaceutical industry has the rights to patent products as well as processes throughout the world, including India. This has led to a significant growth of the pharmaceutical industry, both domestically in India and globally, including increased stakes of multi-national companies in Indian operations.

As a signatory to the WTO Agreements, India is looked upon as a favorable destination for conducting global clinical trials. India clearly provides an opportunity in terms of availability of large patient populations, highly educated talent, English speaking doctors, wide spectrum of disease, lower cost of operations and favorable economic and IP environment *etc.* The overall time and cost advantage in bringing a drug to the market by leveraging India's resources could be as high as US$ 200 million. This is evident by steadily increasing number of global studies in India over past 2 years. Major pharmaceutical companies estimate the total market for conducting clinical trials either directly or through contract research organizations in India through 2010 at US$ 2 billion. Contract Research Organizations (CRO) themselves are fast gaining importance because of their global presence, specialized local expertise as well as competitive pricing strategies and a significant number of new CROs have set up their operations in India over the past few years.

However, some key barriers stand in way of opportunities that includes patient's rights and safety, regulatory framework, infrastructure, ethics committees, data quality, lack of training curriculums on clinical research etc. Most of these barriers are common to all developing countries and needs to be addressed in a similar way[1].

Because the clinical investigator plays a major role in the ethical conduct of any clinical trial. The successful outcome of any clinical trial depends on how the investigator(s) has assumed his overall responsibility. Most of the barriers mentioned above can be easily addressed if a clinical investigator is committed towards ethical conduct of trials.

A segment of ideologues in India believe that clinical trials conduct poses a serious threat to the society because of issues realted to patient's rights and safety, regulatory compliance, unethical trials, infrastructure and training issues as well as exorbitant drug pricing. Following points explain that all these perceived threats are just perceptions, not reality.

Patient's Rights and Safety

In today's scientific era, research is taking major strides in multiple areas to develop new and better drugs to cure ailments that are difficult to treat. In a majority of cases, these drugs are aimed at providing answers to unmet medical needs. However, the drug development process requires 10 to 12 years on average to reach the marketing approval stage.

Participation in clinical trials provides an opportunity to experience the benefits of these new drugs. So a critically ill patient who participates in a clinical trial, and who may not be alive after 8 to 10 years when the drug would be made available in the market, has access to what may provide either longer term health benefits or an improved quality of life. By carefully evaluating the eligibility criteria, a clinical investigator can offer new hope to patients across a wide range of therapeutic areas.

Participation in clinical trials also provides research professionals opportunities to offer the best care to patients. A well-designed and executed study has built-in provisions to ensure patient rights and safety. In fact, a patient may be far safer in a clinical trial than in routine medical care because careful observations are made on safety (toxicity) and efficacy.

In addition, clinical trials move in phases, that is, Phase II trials are initiated only if the Phase I results are promising. Similarly, Phase III trials are conducted only if the drug has shown required safety and efficacy in early phase trials. Hence, a patient is at minimized risk during later phases of clinical trials. In contrast, historical events like the sulfanilamide[2] and thalidomide[3] disasters could have been avoided with appropriate clinical trials. This phase process is particularly important in developing countries if carefully understood and explained to potential subjects.

Regulatory Framework

Multinational pharmaceutical companies and CROs are able to conduct good quality clinical trials in India despite infrastructural challenges at the regulatory department level. They can do so because of required professional training and the professionals' willingness to comply with regulations and applicable standards in a spirit that protects the rights and safety of trial subjects. In India, no less than in the rest of the world, it is the responsibility of individual stakeholders (sponsors, CROs, investigators) to observe self-discipline while conducting clinical trials, especially when there are more than 20,000 big and small companies and a mere handful of regulatory professionals.

The belief that compliance with Good Clinical Practices (GCP) and applicable regulatory guidelines requires the presence of a robust regulatory inspection system is erroneous. Rather, what may be required is a change of mindset from one of "situational ethics" (that is, compliance with medical ethics in clinical trials only) to one of "holistic ethics" (that is, compliance with medical ethics in clinical trials as well as routine medical care). No regulatory authority can ensure 100% GCP compliance unless the individual stakeholders are willing to comply with the applicable regulations.

Conduct of Illegal/Unethical Trials

Scientific misconduct is a global phenomenon linked to human behavior rather than to an individual country. For instance, the U.S. Food and Drug Administration (FDA) website lists the details of clinical investigators who have been "disqualified" or "restricted" from doing research on grounds of scientific misconduct.[4,5] Details of warning letters issued to various stakeholders (clinical investigator, ERB/IRB, sponsor, CRO, *etc.*) can also be obtained from the same website. However, FDA has not banned clinical trials based on these grounds, these individuals, or individual organizations. Rather, FDA has increased its surveillance over clinical research programs. In like manner, the Indian regulatory authority is also in the process of setting up surveillance teams for ensuring ethical conduct of clinical trials.

Companies acting ethically set globally consistent standards and conduct trials only in the countries where GCP compliance is assured. Indian investigators have demonstrated their compliance by virtue of participation in more than 60 global trials so far. Moreover, a majority of those trials were FDA or European registration trials, requiring strict compliance with GCP and regulatory guidelines. The data have been accepted by foreign regulatory authorities and published in international scientific journals of repute.

Infrastructure

Participation in global clinical trials requires an upgrade in existing infrastructure and facilities at a majority of Indian hospitals in terms of functioning of ERB/IRB, calibration and quality control of diagnostic equipments, maintenance of patient medical records, handling of investigational product, and other critical areas.

There have been instances of sponsors providing highly expensive diagnostic instruments to trial sites in order to achieve consistency in trial data globally. All the trials include investigator grants and funding that is generally utilized to upgrade the infrastructure and education facilities at a site. The Institutional Ethics Committees at a majority of Indian hospitals are gaining competence in evaluating the trial proposals from scientific and ethical standpoints. This, in turn, is strengthening the healthcare system of the country while bolstering the ability of institutions to conduct research. In short, clinical research offers value and value-added infrastructural incentives to the country.

Training

Lack of technical know how on drug development and the habit of "copying" (mostly producing generic drugs) are the major hurdles for indigenous drug research. Participation in global trials provides learning opportunities to Indian doctors and scientists, which in turn can be utilized to find the answers for the diseases that are endemic to the country, such as kala-azar, leprosy, trachoma, and tuberculosis. The medical research intellectual base of the country has been sub-optimally utilized so far due to the absence of basic research facilities and know how.

Participation of Indian investigators in global trials and subsequent publication/ presentation motivate them to develop research protocols for domestic healthcare issues. This, in turn, is nurturing a culture of medical research that can match international standards.

Pricing

Less than 10% by value of drugs used in India are of the premium category; the other 90% are established off-patent drugs (drugs for which multiple generic versions are available). Even for premium category drugs, the pricing is generally moderated by three important factors:

> ➢ the purchasing power of the customers;

> ➢ the existence of unpatented drugs and cheaper substitutes; and

> ➢ the Drug Price Control Order, which regulates the pricing of essential life-saving drugs in India.

Even today, people who can afford the premium category drugs are getting them imported from the West or are traveling to other countries to get better medical care. The availability of such drugs in India is going to reduce the overall healthcare cost.

Conclusion

Although it typically takes 10 to 12 years and millions of dollars to bring one new drug to market, the success rate is small. In the developing world, no company or institute wants to, or can, invest such time and resources for a marginal improvement in responses over existing therapies. Fortunately, in a majority of cases, clinical trials can provide answers regarding the use of a therapeutic agent that can benefit millions of patients worldwide. Being the second most populated country in the world, India can contribute significantly to global drug development programs. The foundation of knowledge-based industries in India was laid down by the information technology industry, and there is no reason why clinical research cannot follow in those footsteps. Indian investigators and clinical research professionals have already demonstrated their medical and scientific skills by participating in multiple global clinical trials. It is time now to move forward to capitalize on the opportunity.

References

1. Fenn CG,Wong E, and Zambrano D. 2001. The contemporary situation for the conduct of clinical trials in Asia. International Journal of Pharmaceutical Medicine 15: 169-73.

2. Wax PM. 1995. Elixirs, diluents, and the passage of the 1938 Federal Food, Drug and Cosmetic Act. Annals of Internal Medicine 122: 456-61.

3. Diggle GE. 2001. Thalidomide: 40 years on. International Journal of Pharmaceutical Medicine 55: 627-31.

4. U.S. Food and Drug Administration. Disqualified/Restricted/Assurance List for Clinical Investigators.
   Available from: www.fda.gov/ora/ compliance_ref/bimo/dis_res_assur.htm.

5. U.S. Food and Drug Administration. Disqualified or Totally Restricted List for Clinical Investigators. Available from: www.fda.gov/ora/compliance_ref/bimo/ disqlist.htm.

Appendix-5. Undertaking by the Investigator

(Appendix VII Schedule-Y Rule 122 Drugs and Cosmetics Act, 1945)

1.	Full name, address and title of the Principal Investigator (or Investigator(s) when there is no Principal Investigator)
2.	Name and address of the medical college, hospital or other facility where the clinical trial will be conducted:
3.	Education, training & experience that qualify the Investigator for the clinical trial (Attach details including Medical Council registration number, and / or any other statement(s) of qualification(s)) ☐ Curriculum Vitae ☐ Other Statement of Qualifications
4.	Name and address of all clinical laboratory facilities to be used in the study.
5.	Name and address of the Ethics Committee that is responsible for approval and continuing review of the study.
6.	Names of the other members of the research team (Co- or sub-Investigators) who will be assisting the Investigator in the conduct of the investigation (s).
7.	Protocol Title and Study number (if any) of the clinical trial to be conducted by the Investigator.
8.	Commitments:
(i)	I have reviewed the clinical protocol and agree that it contains all the necessary information to conduct the study. I will not begin the study until all necessary Ethics Committee and regulatory approvals have been obtained.
(ii)	I agree to conduct the study in accordance with the current protocol. I will not implement any deviation from or changes of the protocol without agreement by the Sponsor and prior review and documented approval / favorable opinion from the Ethics Committee of the amendment, except where necessary to eliminate an immediate hazard(s) to the trial Subjects or when the change(s) involved are only logistical or administrative in nature.

(iii) I agree to personally conduct and/or supervise the clinical trial at my site.

(iv) I agree to inform all Subjects, that the drugs are being used for investigational purposes and I will ensure that the requirements relating to obtaining informed consent and ethics committee review and approval specified in the GCP guidelines are met.

(v) I agree to report to the Sponsor all adverse experiences that occur in the course of the investigation(s) in   accordance with the regulatory and GCP guidelines.

(vi) I have read and understood the information in the Investigator's brochure, including the potential risks and side effects of the drug.

(vii) I agree to ensure that all associates, colleagues and employees assisting in the conduct of the study are suitably qualified and experienced and they have been informed about their obligations in meeting their commitments in the trial.

(viii) I agree to maintain adequate and accurate records and to make those records available for audit / inspection by the Sponsor, Ethics Committee, Licensing Authority or their authorized representatives, in accordance with regulatory and GCP provisions. I will fully cooperate with any study related audit conducted by regulatory officials or authorized representatives of the Sponsor.

(ix) I agree to promptly report to the Ethics Committee all changes in the clinical trial activities and all unanticipated problems involving risks to human Subjects or others.

(x) I agree to inform all unexpected serious adverse events to the Sponsor as well as the Ethics Committee within seven days of their occurrence.

(xi) I will maintain confidentiality of the identification of all participating study patients and assure security and confidentiality of study data.

(xii) I agree to comply with all other requirements, guidelines and statutory obligations as applicable to clinical Investigators participating in clinical trials.

9. Signature of Investigator   10. Date

www.ingramcontent.com/pod-product-compliance
Lightning Source LLC
Chambersburg PA
CBHW070723220326
41598CB00024BA/3279